EMINENT DOCTORS.

EMINENT DOCTORS:

𝕿𝖍𝖊𝖎𝖗 𝕷𝖎𝖛𝖊𝖘 𝖆𝖓𝖉 𝖙𝖍𝖊𝖎𝖗 𝖂𝖔𝖗𝖐.

BY

GEORGE T. BETTANY

"There is to me an inexpressible charm in the lives of the good, brave, learned men, whose only objects have been, and are, to alleviate pain and to save life."
—G. A. SALA.

IN TWO VOLUMES.

VOL. I.

Essay Index Reprint Series

BOOKS FOR LIBRARIES PRESS
FREEPORT, NEW YORK

First Published 1885
Reprinted 1972

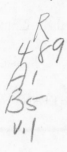

Library of Congress Cataloging in Publication Data

Bettany, George Thomas, 1850-1891.
   Eminent doctors.

   (Essay index reprint series)
   Reprint of the 1885 ed.
   1. Physicians--Gt. Brit. 2. Medicine--Gt. Brit.
--History. I. Title.
R489.A1B5 1972   610'.922 [B]   76-39663
ISBN 0-8369-2747-8

PRINTED IN THE UNITED STATES OF AMERICA
BY
NEW WORLD BOOK MANUFACTURING CO., INC.
HALLANDALE, FLORIDA 33009

PREFACE.

MEDICAL Biography has not taken its due place in the thoughts of our countrymen, nor has it received deserved attention from literary men. Anecdotes of big fees, brilliant operations, brusque actions, or suave politeness, have too exclusively contributed to form the popular idea of eminent physicians and surgeons. Aikin's incomplete "Biographical Memoirs of Medicine," Macmichael's "Lives of British Physicians," and Pettigrew's "Medical Portrait Gallery," have been the chief collective records of British medical men; and the latter, owing to its expensive form, was inaccessible to most persons. Munk's "Roll of the College of Physicians" is a mine of information about members of that College, and a similar record of members of the College of Surgeons would be invaluable. In 1865 Dr. Herbert Barker commenced, and after

his lamented death Dr. Tindal Robertson continued, a series of memoirs of living medical
men, accompanied by photographs. The *Mid-
land Medical Miscellany* commenced to publish
a somewhat similar series of memoirs, with
portraits, in 1882. The medical press has
been distinguished for the ability and general
fidelity of its biographical notices of deceased
members of the profession.

There is no book, however, in current literature which supplies medical men or the general
public with biographical accounts of the most
notable men who in this kingdom have contributed to make the medicine and surgery of
to-day what they are. It is the aim of the
present book to occupy this vacant place. It
is hoped that this has been done in a form
neither too technical for the general reader, nor
unsuitable for the busy practitioner, who has
very little time to read elaborate biographies,
but would fain store his mind with the principal
facts and lessons of the lives of his great predecessors and teachers.

The difficulty of selection has been great.
It was felt that sure ground would be occupied
by taking the foundation of the London College

of Physicians as a starting-point, and giving a place only to those celebrated men in the seventeenth and eighteenth centuries whose title to fame none would deny. Paucity of biographical materials has prevented the introduction of some names; others have been excluded because they were rather notorious for their fees, their *bonmots*, or their fantastic behaviour, than for their solid contributions to medicine.

In regard to men of the present century, the task of selection has been still more difficult. For the most part distinguished physiologists, zoologists, &c., do not find a place in these pages, unless they have also won distinction in medical practice. It cannot be expected that the list of living names will satisfy everybody. Others as worthy might have been included. If in refraining from commenting on the career of his present colleagues at Guy's Hospital, the author may appear to have done injustice to their great merits, he is convinced that he has thereby best steered clear of the dangers of partiality. The utmost care has been taken to avoid giving details which should be private during a man's life, and to state only those facts about living men which have already for the most part been made generally accessible.

The task of reading hundreds of biographical memoirs, medical treatises, scattered pamphlets and papers, has been exceedingly heavy. All those named in the following pages have been consulted; and where details are not given of controversies or incidents which some may be surprised to see passed over, this has been the result of careful deliberation. The author desires specially to acknowledge his great obligations to the *Lancet* and other medical journals. He trusts he has contributed to the object which they, like himself, have at heart, of elevating the medical profession in the public estimation.

DULWICH, *September* 1885.

CONTENTS OF VOL. I.

CONTENTS OF VOL.

EMINENT DOCTORS.

CHAPTER I.

LINACRE, CAIUS, AND THE FOUNDATION OF BRITISH MEDICINE.

THE name of THOMAS LINACRE must stand at the head of any account of the history of British medicine, for before his accession to the office of tutor and physician to Prince Arthur, eldest son of Henry VII., in 1501, no physician of such ability as to have left works of permanent value had arisen in this country. To him belongs the honour of having founded the Royal College of Physicians of London, the earliest of the British medical corporations; and by that one act he may be said to have constituted medicine a distinct profession. The slightness of the emphasis which can be laid upon the medical profession up to Linacre's time may be recognised from the fact that he was both tutor and medical attendant to a prince, and that he subsequently became a not undistinguished ecclesiastic.

Canterbury gave birth to this founder of British

A

medicine about 1460. He derived his descent, however, from a Derbyshire family of Saxon blood flourishing before the Conquest at Linacre, near Chesterfield. His schooldays were passed under the superintendence of William Selling, at the monastic school of Christchurch in Canterbury. Selling was an enlightened man for his time, and had travelled in Italy, where he studied Greek with one of the most eager students of the time, Politian, and had brought home with him numerous valuable manuscripts. A fellow of All Souls' himself, he doubtless had some influence in securing the election of his pupil to a fellowship there at an early age, in 1484. At Oxford Linacre was a pupil of Cornelio Vitelli, an Italian, one of the earliest teachers who brought Greek learning into this country.

Before long Linacre himself took charge of pupils, the most **famous** of whom afterwards became Sir Thomas More. Linacre accompanied Selling to Italy when Henry VII. appointed the latter on a mission to the Roman pontiff. In Italy he received the benefit of introductions to, and instructions from, Politian and others, and formed an acquaintance with Aldus Manutius, the celebrated printer, at Venice. At Florence he was introduced to Lorenzo de Medici, who specially approved of his companionship with his sons both in their studies and their amusements. After taking the degree of Doctor of Medicine in the University of Padua with great applause, owing to the skill with which he defended the positions of his thesis, he returned to England. He apparently betook himself at once to Oxford, where he was incorporated M.D. It is presumed that he was still most concerned in academical pursuits; and he was the first Englishman to publish a correct rendering of a Greek author after the revival of letters, namely, the "Sphere" of Proclus, printed by Aldus at Venice in 1499. Whether he was also incorporated at Cambridge, as Dr. Caius relates, cannot now be proved, but it is rendered probable by the fact of his subsequent foundation of a lectureship in medicine at that university.

At this period of his life Linacre had the good fortune to be the instructor, especially in Greek, of no less a person than Erasmus. The latter was evidently a most appreciative admirer of our erudite doctor, as well as of the facilities for classical study afforded in England. "In Colet," says he, writing to Robert Fisher, "I hear Plato himself. Who does not admire the perfect compass of science in Grocyn? Is aught more acute, more exalted, or more refined than the judgment of Linacre? Has nature framed anything either milder, sweeter, or happier than the disposition of More? It is wonderful how universally copious is here the harvest of ancient learning, wherefore you should hasten your return."

With the beginning of the sixteenth century, however, a new era in Linacre's life dawns. Whether or not he was introduced to court in 1501 in connection with the visit of Prince Arthur to Oxford, it is certain

that about the period when the prince was contracted
in marriage to Catherine of Arragon, his health and
further education were intrusted to Dr. Linacre; and
it is believed, though without sure grounds, that he
also became one of the king's domestic physicians.

The death of the young prince, however, relieving
Linacre of his tutorial duties, appears to have had the
effect of throwing him with ardent zeal into the practice
of the medical profession. Erasmus had availed himself of his skill, as is testified by a letter of his from
Paris in 1506, giving an account of his complaints, and
lamenting the want of his accustomed advice and prescriptions. His friends even found that he was too
devoted to his studies and practice, and begged him to
relax so far as to write to them occasionally. Probably
the economical disposition of Henry VII. prevented
Linacre from reaping too great a reward from his connection with the court, and he would hail with hopeful
feelings the accession of Henry VIII. with his more
liberal tendencies. His position was soon assured by
his appointment as one of the king's physicians,
apparently the principal one; and his estimation at
court was higher than his office alone would have
occasioned, in consequence of his learning and social
qualities. His other patients included Cardinal Wolsey,
Archbishop Warham, and Fox, Bishop of Winchester.

About the commencement of Henry VIII.'s reign
Linacre took up the study of theology, which he had
previously neglected in his zeal for the revival of

letters; and, in accordance with the practice of the age, on becoming convinced of the importance of Christian doctrines, he sought ordination. In October 1509 the Primate gave him the rectory of Merstham, in Kent, which he held only a month, receiving in December a prebendal stall in the cathedral of Wells, and in 1510 the cure of Hawkhurst, in Kent, which he held till 1524. Still higher preferment, however, awaited him, for he became canon and prebend of Westminster in 1517. Numerous other appointments followed, which we will not particularise. It does not appear certain that Linacre gained any conspicuous distinction in theology, but his preferments were rather acknowledgments of his general learning and merit, being the most convenient form in which such recognition could at that time be given.

Linacre's intercourse with Erasmus continued, but was somewhat embarrassed by reason of the latter's constant demand for pecuniary aid. We gain a glimpse of the prudence which Linacre had attained, from a letter of Erasmus in 1521, complaining of the unfavourable reception of his applications for money, mentioning that though his health was infirm, and though he possessed only six angels, he had been advised to curtail his expenses and bear his poverty with fortitude, rather than apply further to the Primate and Lord Mountjoy.

We have now to recur to Linacre's medical pursuits, which were not interrupted to any serious extent by his clerical preferments. Early in Henry VIII.'s reign, he read before the University of Oxford a "Shagglyng" lecture, of which nothing but the name is preserved. His renewed connection with Oxford occasioned it to be bruited abroad that he had a special design of making benefactions to the university, and the authorities bethought themselves that they had somewhat neglected their distinguished alumnus. Consequently they presented him with an address, in which they seem to have been actuated by that kind of gratitude which consists in a lively sense of favours to come. Part of it runs thus (translated from Latin), showing how much dignity a learned university then possessed :—

"To Thomas Linacre, the most skilful physician of the king.

"We are not a little troubled, excellent sir (to mention nothing besides), and most learned of physicians, since till now we have never greeted your pre-eminence by letter (let us confess the truth), how we may readily devise the means by which we may handsomely remove from ourselves the stain of ingratitude which we have incurred, were we otherwise than assured that you are rather displeased at the greater goodwill, nay the more ardent affection, which your courtesy has entertained towards our university, than at any negligence, not to say sluggishness of our own. How excellent the mind, how liberal the devotion of him, who, whilst he is the most eminent, is indisputably the most eloquent of his contemporaries, towards the university of Oxford, is a secret to none. How well you think of us, and how generously you have resolved to provide for our interests, we have fully learned from the report of our colleagues, who have discoursed with you. . . . But that we have yet made no returns for your extraordinary bounty towards us (to repay, alas! accords not with our poverty), which we can only do with our whole hearts . . . we give you truly our fullest thanks, resting our chief hope in you, whose reputation stands so high with the king's majesty, that we may with good reason commemorate you amongst the most active leaders and foremost patrons of our academical host."

The form which very many attempts to promote the progress of medicine in that age took was that of translations of and commentaries on the works of Galen, which in the original Greek were inaccessible to nearly every one.

After spending much time on executing his share of a scheme for translating Aristotle's entire works into Latin, in conjunction with Grocyn and Thomas Latimer, and which unfortunately never was published, Dr. Linacre betook himself to the congenial task of translating into Latin Galen's works, the first portion of which, on the Preservation of Health, was published at Paris in 1517, and dedicated to Henry VIII. The feelings which moved him to this act arose, as he declares to the king, from finding himself wanting in the means of vying with those who, allured by the renown and glory of his name, daily contended in the number and variety of their gifts. For this reason he knew nothing more becoming his duty or his calling, than the dedication of some memorial of his studies, that he might satisfactorily account for the leisure which, by the royal indulgence, he sometimes stole from his appointed attendance, and at the same time show that he not only spent the hours of office, but even of recreation from its duties, in accomplishing, to the best of his ability, what he thought would be acceptable to him. A copy of this work on vellum, and magnificently embellished, was presented to Wolsey, with an adulatory letter. These are still preserved in the British Museum.

This translation was followed by several others from Galen, including the Method of Healing, 1519, dedicated to the king; the treatise on Temperaments, 1521, dedicated to Leo X.; on the Natural Functions, 1523, dedicated to Warham; on the Pulse, 1523, dedicated to Wolsey. Other treatises left complete at Linacre's death were printed by Pynson in 1524. Of the treatises on grammar and language, compiled by Linacre, we need not here attempt to give an account.

Most important of all Linacre's achievements towards the advancement of medicine was undoubtedly his securing the foundation of the Royal College of Physicians. "The practice of medicine," says his biographer, Dr. J. N. Johnson, "when this scheme was

carried into effect, was scarcely elevated above that of
the mechanical arts; nor were the majority of its practitioners better educated than mechanics. No society
as yet existed, independent of the monastic and eccle-
siastical, which could at all be considered learned."

Linacre was at the sole expense of founding the
college, for the crown merely granted the letters
patent. These were issued in 1518, incorporating all
physicians in London as one faculty and college, with
power to elect a president, to use a common seal, and
to hold lands not exceeding the annual value of £12.
They were to hold assemblies and govern their faculty
in London and within seven miles, all persons being
interdicted from practice who did not hold their license.
Four censors were to be chosen yearly, for the correction
and government of physic and its professors, the examination of medicines, and the punishment of offenders;
and physicians were to be exempt from attendance at
assizes, inquests, and juries. The power of correction
by fine or imprisonment occasioned some embarrass-
ment at a subsequent period, for when some offenders
were committed by the college, the gaolers would not
receive them into prison, considering the college must
charge itself with the custody of its own culprits. To
obviate this difficulty a statute (1 Mary, sess. 2, c. 9)
was passed, requiring gaolers to receive persons committed by the college, and also enjoining all justices,
mayors, &c., in London to assist the President of the
college in searching for faulty apothecary wares.

Various defects having been found in the original letters patent, they were confirmed by a statute, 14 Henry VIII. (1523), which provided among other things that no person except graduates of Oxford or Cambridge should be permitted to practise physic throughout England, unless examined and approved by the President of the College of Physicians of London, and at least three other selected members. Previous to Linacre's time, the bishops or their vicars-general were the persons who could grant licences to practise medicine (in addition to the universities), and this power was long after this retained by them, although they called in physicians to assist them in determining to whom licences should be granted.

As was but natural, Linacre was the first President of the college which owed its existence to himself, and he held that office till his death. His residence, the Stone House, in Knight-Rider Street, Paul's Wharf, convenient for access to the Court, then kept up at Bridewell, was also the meeting-place of the college. The front portion of the house, a parlour below, and a council room and library above, were given to the college during his lifetime, and remained the property of the college until 1860.

In considering the import of Linacre's endeavours to promote the study of medicine at Oxford and Cambridge, it must be remembered that the idea of establishing lectureships or professorships for public instruction was quite a novel one in England, and that

Fox, Bishop of Winchester, appears to have been the first, in 1517, to endow lectures in Greek and Latin. And Linacre unquestionably has the merit of first applying such an idea to the improvement of instruction in medicine. His foundations did not take full effect till 1524. Again, we have a letter from the University of Oxford " to the renowned Dr. Linacre," couched in the most exaggerated style of panegyric, thanking him for his proposition to endow " splendid lectures " in medicine, lauding his " sober gravity and erudite judgment," " his greatness," " the transcendency of his gifts." The letters patent founding the lectures were dated on the 12th of October, 1524, only eight days before his death. Two of the lectureships were to be founded at Oxford and one at Cambridge, and to be named Linacre's Lectures. Thirty pounds a year, a considerable sum then, was to be devoted to this purpose by his trustees, out of the proceeds of two manors at Newington, near Sittingbourne. But although the trustees, Sir Thomas More, Tonstal, Stokesley, Tonstal's successor, and John Shelley, were men who might have been expected to pay attention to Linacre's desires, yet, probably owing to the busy occupations in which they were engaged, they failed to carry them into full effect; and it was not till the third year of Edward VI. that Tonstal, the surviving trustee, assigned two of the lecturers to Merton College, Oxford, and one to St. John's College, Cambridge. Their office was to expound publicly certain parts of Hippocrates or Galen. That his lectures failed to become what Linacre would have wished, was due to the common defect of that age in not foreseeing the revolutions in learning that were to come, and not providing any elasticity in their foundations. Thus these lectureships, which might have powerfully aided the development of medicine, remained of little use till modern times, when they have been placed on an improved footing.

"It has been questioned," writes his biographer, "whether he was a better Latinist or Grecian, a better grammarian or physician, a better scholar or man. That Linacre was of a great natural sagacity, and of a discerning judgment in his own profession, we have the concurrent testimony of the most knowing of his contemporaries. In many cases which were considered desperate, his practice was successful. In the case of his friend Lilye, he foretold his certain death if he submitted to the opinion of some rash persons who advised him and prevailed with him to have a malignant strumous tumour in his hip cut off, and his prognostic was justified by the event.

"In private life he had an utter detestation of everything that was dishonourable; he was a faithful friend, and was valued and beloved by all ranks in life. He showed a remarkable kindness to young students in his profession; and those whom he found distinguished for ingenuity, modesty, learning, good manners, or a desire to excel, he assisted with his advice, his interest, and his purse."

Linacre had suffered for years from stone in the bladder, which had limited his usefulness and the perfection of several of his designs; and he died of ulceration of the bladder, on the 20th October, 1524, having made his will four months previously. He was buried in St. Paul's Cathedral, in a spot chosen by himself, and expressly named in his will. No memorial was erected over his grave until 1557, when Dr. Caius, one of his successors, reared a monument with a suitable inscription, ending with a favourite expression which he afterwards placed on his own tomb, "Vivit post funera virtus."

The will of Dr. Linacre includes annuities to his two sisters, a bequest to his brother, and other legacies. To his nieces Alice and Margaret he bequeathed each a bed, Margaret to have the better; and to William Dancaster, a priest who witnessed the will, a feather-bed and two Irish blankets were left. The simplicity of these details shows that a man of high distinction in many ways at that time counted as important possessions articles now universal.*

JOHN KAYE or KEY, better known by the Latinised form CAIUS, which retains nevertheless the pronunciation derived from the English original, Keys, was born at Norwich on the 6th of October, 1510, being thus fourteen years old at Linacre's death. He entered

---

* Life of Thomas Linacre. By J. Noble Johnson, M. D. London. 1835.

Gonville Hall, Cambridge, on the 12th September, 1529, and here he early distinguished himself by translating from Greek into Latin two treatises—one by Chrysostom—and by making an abridgment of Erasmus's "De Verâ Theologiâ." He took the degree of B.A. in 1532-3, and was appointed principal of Physwick Hostel on the 12th November, 1533, being elected to a fellowship of Gonville Hall on December 6th following. Proceeding M.A. in 1535, he is recorded as subscribing, with the master and fellows of Gonville Hall, the submission to Henry VIII.'s injunctions.

In 1539 he went to Italy, and studied medicine at Padua under Montanus, lodging in the same house with Vesalius, who became the most distinguished anatomist of his time. In 1541 the degree of Doctor of Medicine was conferred upon him at Padua, where in the next year we find him delivering public lectures on the Greek text of Aristotle, in conjunction with Realdus Columbus, the stipend for which was provided by some Venetian nobles. The next year, 1543, he largely occupied in visiting all the most celebrated libraries of Italy, collating manuscripts, principally with a view to publishing correct editions of Galen and Celsus.

Returning to England after further travels in France and Germany, he was incorporated M.D. at Cambridge, and practised apparently at Cambridge, Norwich, and Shrewsbury, with such success that he was appointed physician to Edward VI., an appointment he continued to hold under Queens Mary and Elizabeth. On the

22d December, 1547, he was admitted a Fellow of the College of Physicians, and in 1550 became an Elect, in 1552 Censor. In the latter year appeared his English treatise on the Sweating Sickness, which had broken out at Shrewsbury in 1551. This was afterwards enlarged and published in Latin.

"The Boke or Counseill against the Sweatyng Sicknesse," was dedicated by Dr. Caius to William, Earl of Pembroke. The dedication begins thus : " In the fearful time of the sweat, many resorted unto me for counsel, among whom some being my friends and acquaintance, desired me to write unto them some little counsel how to govern themselves therein. . . . At whose request at that time, I wrote divers counsels so shortly as I could for the present necessity, which they both used and did give abroad to many others, and further appointed in myself to fulfil the other part of their honest request for the time to come. The which the better to execute and bring to pass, I spared not to go to all those that sent for me, both poor and rich, day and night. And that not only to do them that ease that I could, and to instruct them for their recovery ; but to note also thoroughly the cases and circumstances of the disease in divers persons, and to understand the nature and causes of the same fully, for so much as might be."

A certain conceit is evident throughout the brief treatise, as when he describes his early translations from Latin into English, and partially apologises for writing in English, then gives an account of the life and writings of his friend, William Framingham, a fellow-townsman of his who died young. The description of the disease which he gives indicates a very acute rheumatic affection, inasmuch as perspirations of disagreeable odour, acute pains in the limbs, delirium, quick and irritable pulse, &c., were prominent among them.

It is notable how little medical science was progressing beyond Galenic principles. Dr. Caius says, " This disease is not a sweat only, but a fever in the spirits by putrefaction venomous, with a fight, travail, and labour of nature against the infection received in the spirits, whereupon by chance followeth a sweat, or issueth an humour, compelled by nature, as also chanceth in other sicknesses which consist in humours." Still, a glimpse of truth is shown in the view expressed that " our bodies can not suffer anything or hurt by corrupt and infective causes, except there be in them a certain matter prepared, apt and like to receive it, else if one were sick, all should be sick."

Dr. Caius showed himself notably before his age also in his censures of excess in eating and drinking, his commendation of the bath, and of muscular exercise His advice to his readers to have recourse to a good physician, and to be at least as good to their bodies as to their hose or their shoes, is followed by a picture of the army of quacks who in default of science preyed upon the masses. " Simple-women, carpenters, pewterers, braziers, soapball-sellers, apothecaries, avaunters themselves to come from Pole, Constantinople, Italy, Almaine, Spain, France, Greece, Turkey, India, Egypt or Jury; from the service of emperors, kings, and queens, promising help of all diseases, yea incurable, with one or two drinks, by drinks of great and high prices, as though they were made of the sun, moon, or stars, by blessings and blowings, hypocritical prayings, and foolish smokings of shirts, smocks, and kerchiefs, with such others, their phantasies and mockeries, meaning nothing else but to abuse your light belief, and scorn you behind your backs, with their medicines (so filthy, that I am ashamed to name them), for your single wit and simple belief, in trusting them most, which you know not at all, and understand least; like to them which think far fowls have fair feathers, although they be never so evil favoured and foul; as though there could not be so cunning an Englishman, as a foolish running stranger, or so perfect health by honest learning, as by deceitful ignorance." From all which the reader may judge whether somewhat similar remarks might not be applicable to the last century, and even to a great part of the present, in its credulity of the efficacy of quack medicines and the powers of audacious empirics.

In 1555 Dr. Caius was elected President of the College of Physicians, an office which he continued to hold until 1561. He applied himself with devoted energy to promoting the interests of the college, commencing to record its annals, till then unpreserved, procuring the copying and binding in grand style of the college statutes, designing the insignia, the cushion of crimson velvet edged with gold on which the statutes were laid, the silver staff ornamented with the college arms borne by the President, to remind him, according to Caius, by its material (silver), to govern with patience and courtesy, and by its symbols (the serpents), with judgment and wisdom. His zeal further exhibited itself in protecting the privileges of the college, as when he appeared successfully, in Elizabeth's reign, against the barber surgeons, who were claiming the right to prescribe medicines for internal administration in cases where their operative assistance was called in.

One of the most striking innovations which Dr. Caius introduced into this country was unquestionably the practice of dissection of the human body. He had actually taught practical anatomy in the Barber Surgeons' Hall, not long after his return from Italy; and he further provided for the development of that science by procuring from Queen Elizabeth, about 1564, a grant to the College of Physicians to take annually the bodies of two criminals after execution, for dissection, and the fellows were required, under penalty of a fine for refusing, to give demonstrations and lectures on anatomy in turn. He left a fund for defraying the expenses attending these dissections.

Dr. Caius had never wavered in his attachment to

learning, and to his alma mater, Cambridge. Notwithstanding his numerous public interests, the court, the
college, and private practice, he developed fully and
had the pleasure of carrying into execution a design for
improving and enlarging Gonville Hall, which under
his auspices became a college, with the addition of his
name to its title. He added to its resources very considerably, founded three fellowships and twenty scholar-
ships, and enlarged it by building an entirely new court,
known as Caius Court. Together with this enlargement he pleased his taste by erecting three new gates,
two on its external boundaries, and one within it. The
first, severely simple, was inscribed "Humilitatis;" the
second, more lofty, and surmounted by several rooms,
was on one side inscribed "Virtutis," on the other
"Jo. Caius posuit Sapientiæ." The last, smaller, but
highly decorated, leading to the Senate House and the
Schools, bore the word "Honoris;" and thus the worthy
doctor signified that by way of humility we attain to
virtue and honour.

By the authority of letters patent granted by Philip
and Mary, 4th September, 1557, Dr. Caius was
authorised to frame new statutes for Gonville and
Caius College. It was not till 1558 that he was incorporated M.D. at Cambridge, and the next January he
was reluctantly induced to accept the dignity of master
of the college, which then fell vacant. He made this a
further occasion of benefaction by refusing the stipend
and emoluments of the office, which he held till one

month before his death. For one year he resigned the presidency of the College of Physicians, that he might more uninterruptedly superintend the erection of his new court at Cambridge; but he returned to the presidency for 1562–3, and again in 1571.

A man of Dr. Caius's incessant activity and zeal for his own opinions could not hope to remain without enemies. In 1565 three fellows of his college, whom he had expelled, charged him with atheism and opposition to professors of the Gospel. His maintenance of his post at court under sovereigns of opposite religious professions, notwithstanding his attachment to Romanism, was made a subject of accusation of unsteadiness in his religious principles. Fuller remarks that "his being a reputed papist was no great crime to such who consider the time when he was born, and foreign places wherein he was bred. However, this I dare say in his just defence: he never mentioneth Protestants but with due respect, and sometimes doth occasionally condemn the superstitious credulity of popish miracles." Nevertheless, he retained in his college certain books and vestments formerly used in the Roman Catholic service, and Bishop Sandys having written to the vice-chancellor, Dr. Byng, complaining of this, they were collected and burnt in 1572 (Dec. 13), much to Dr. Caius's vexation, who considered Dr. Byng's action most arbitrary, and inveighed strongly against the conduct of certain fellows of his college in the matter.

Previous to this time, in 1570, Dr. Caius had pub-

lished an account of British dogs, which is the earliest
scientific description of the kind of dogs then occurring
in this country. It had been the result of a request
by the celebrated naturalist, Gesner, whose death in
1565 prevented its earlier publication. Numerous
other accounts of British natural history had been furnished by Dr. Caius to Gesner, and were inserted in
his works. To give an idea of our doctor's ability in
descriptive natural history, we subjoin his account "Of
the dog called a Bloodhound."

"The greater sort which serve to hunt, having lips of
a large size, and ears of no small length, do not only
chase the beast while it liveth, but being dead also by
any manner of casualty, make recourse to the place
where it lieth, having in this point an assured and
infallible guide, namely the scent and savour of the
blood sprinkled here and there upon the ground. For
whether the beast being wounded, doth notwithstanding
enjoy life, and escapeth the hands of the huntsman, or
whether the said beast being slain is conveyed cleanly
out of the park (so that there be some signification of
blood shed), these dogs with no less facility and easi-
ness than avidity and greediness, can disclose and
bewray the same by smelling, applying to their pursuit agility and nimbleness without tediousness. And
albeit peradventure it may chance that a piece of flesh
be subtilly stolen and cunningly conveyed away with
such provisos and precaveats as thereby all appearance
of blood is either prevented, excluded, or concealed, yet

these kind of dogs by a certain direction of an inward assured notice and privy mark, pursue the deed-doers, through long lanes, crooked reaches, and weary ways, without wandering awry out of the limits of the land whereon those desperate purloiners prepared their speedy passage. Yea, the nature of these dogs is such, and so effectual is their foresight, that they can bewray, separate, and pick them out from among an infinite multitude and an innumerable company—creep they never so far into the thickest throng, they will find him out notwithstanding he lie hidden in wild woods, in close and overgrown groves, and lurk in hollow holes apt to harbour such ungracious guests. Moreover, although they should pass over the water, thinking thereby to avoid the pursuit of the hounds, yet will not these dogs give over their attempt, but presuming to swim through the stream, persevere in their pursuit, and when they be arrived and gotten the furthen bank, they hunt up and down, to and fro run they, from place to place shift they, until they have attained to that plot of ground where they passed over."

This treatise was so highly esteemed by Pennant that he inserted it in his British Zoology; and it was reprinted in a very neat form in 1880.*

We need not particularise the very numerous editions and translations from Galen, Celsus, Hippocrates, which Dr. Caius published or left in manuscript. His own original medical works were the Method of Healing,

---

* " Of Englishe Dogges : " 170 Strand, W.C.

based however upon Galen and Montanus, and the
account of the sweating sickness, concerning which
Hecker remarks, "Although, judged according to a
modern standard, it is far from satisfactory, yet it contains an abundance of valuable matter, and proves its
author to be a good observer." *

Dr. Caius is credited with having predicted the very
day of his death. He had his own grave prepared in
Caius College Chapel, on the 2d, 3d, and 4th of July,
1573, and died at his London house on the 29th of the
same month, aged sixty-three. His body being removed
to Cambridge as he had directed, the master and fellows
of his college and the principal members of the university in procession met it at Trumpington. The inscription on his tomb in Caius Chapel is characteristic of
the man, in whose eyes his own works and achievements, undoubtedly considerable, loomed large. " Vivit
post funera virtus," as he had recorded on Linacre's
monument. "Fui Caius," he adds, as a pithy if ego-
tistic comment.

Among other notable men of the sixteenth century
must be mentioned WILLIAM GILBERT, M.D., a native
of Colchester, who was born in 1540, and became
senior fellow of St. John's College, Cambridge, in 1569.
Having settled in London in 1573, his distinction was
such that he became physician to Queen Elizabeth.

* "Epidemics of the Middle Ages." Sydenham Soc. Publ. London
1844.

But he was one of the first of the illustrious series of
English physicians who employed their leisure in philosophical research.   By his book, " On the Magnet, on
Magnetic Bodies, and the Great Magnet the Earth," published in 1600, he had the good fortune to become the
stimulator of Galileo himself to the study of magnetism,
and that master described him as "great to a degree
which might be envied."   Queen Elizabeth added to
her titles to regard by conferring a pension on Gilbert,
which aided him in prosecuting his experiments.   Gilbert was in fact a great originator in science, having
discovered the earth's magnetism, and that to this is
due both the direction of the magnetic needle north
and south, and the variation and dipping of the needle.
Thus he stands as the discoverer of the facts on which
the science of magnetism was based.   He is said to
have been no less exact in chemistry, but unfortunately
nothing of his is extant on that subject.   Fuller says
of him in the " Worthies "—" Mahomet's tomb at Mecca
is said strangely to hang up, attracted by some invisible
loadstone ; but the memory of this doctor will never
fall to the ground, which his incomparable book, ' *De
Magnete,*' will support to eternity."   Gilbert died in 1603,
shortly after being appointed physician to James I.

CHAPTER II.

WILLIAM HARVEY AND THE CIRCULATION OF THE BLOOD.

" Oft have I seen a timely-parted ghost,
  Of ashy semblance, meagre, pale, and bloodless,
  Being all descended to the labouring heart,
  Who in the conflict that he holds with death,
  Attracts the same for aidance 'gainst the enemy ;
  Which with the heart there cools, and ne'er returneth
  To blush and beautify the cheek again."

IF the man who discovered a new material world deserves immortality, equally meritorious is he who
revealed a new world of activity, and promulgated the
first true conception of the ceaseless round of vital processes. As Dr. Parkes says in his Harveian Oration,
1876, "When any one examines into this discovery of
Harvey's, and gradually recognises its extraordinary
importance, he cannot but be seized with an urgent
wish to know how the mind which solved so great a
problem was constituted ; how it worked and how it
reached, not merely the probability, but the certainty,
of a grand natural law. . . . There was no accident
about it—no help from what we call chance ; it was

worked out and thought out, point after point, until all was clear as sunshine in midsummer. Nor had it been anticipated."

WILLIAM HARVEY, eldest son of Thomas Harvey and Joan Halke, was born at Folkestone in Kent, on the 1st of April, 1578, and that his parents were in easy circumstances may be judged by the fact that five of his brothers became substantial London merchants. Of his mother it is recorded on her monumental tablet that she was " a careful, tender-hearted mother, dear to her husband, reverenced of her children, beloved of her neighbours." Her eldest son, after some years' education at Canterbury, was entered at Gonville and Caius College in 1593, where he remained till 1597, when he left the university with the B.A. degree, and betook himself to Padua. This renowned university then boasted among its professors Fabricius, the ana- tomist, whose influence upon Harvey was evidently remarkable. After five years, Harvey obtained his doctorate in medicine, couched in terms of the utmost praise of his astonishing ability, memory, and know- ledge, and returned to England. He was admitted to the same degree at Cambridge, and settled in practice in London, marrying the daughter of Dr. Launcelot Browne in his twenty-sixth year—a union which proved childless.

Having become a candidate for the Fellowship of the College of Physicians in 1604, he was admitted in 1607 after due probation; and we find him in 1609 seeking the reversion of the physiciancy to St. Bartholomew's Hospital, gaining the king's letters recommendatory, and producing such testimonials from the President of the College of Physicians and others that he was chosen before the vacancy occurred, and on the death of Dr. Wilkinson was appointed to the office, October 14, 1609.

Harvey now rapidly advanced in general favour as a physician, and in 1615 was appointed Lumleian Lecturer at the College of Physicians, an office then held for life. His first lectures were given in April 1616, and in this and subsequent years he gradually unfolded the novel views on the heart and the circulation of the blood which he was acquiring, and which he published in 1628. The novelty of his views does not, however, consist in the idea that the blood actually moves in the vessels. This was known before, and Shakespeare gives expression to a current conception in the passage at the head of this chapter. Servetus, in 1553,* had asserted that the blood finds access from the right side of the heart to the left through the lungs, thus explaining the intermixture in the heart of the two kinds of blood appropriate to arteries and veins respectively. For a long time the partition between the ventricles was believed to be perforated like a sieve, so that a mixture of venous and arterial blood could take place. But this had been completely disproved by Berengarius and Vesalius. Consequently

* Restitutio Christianismi.

the two kinds of blood, according to this view, after meeting in the head, thorax, and abdomen, returned to the heart by the way they came, for a fresh supply of the exhausted or enfeebled spirits on which the principal functions of the body depended. Servetus, it is true, asserts a communication between the pulmonary artery and veins; but he particularly declares that " the vital spirit has its origin in the left ventricle, the lungs assisting especially in its generation," and that " it is engendered from the mixture that takes place in the lungs of the inspired air with the elaborated subtile blood which the right ventricle of the heart communicates to the left." The extent of his knowledge is further shown by his statement that " the blood is mixed in the pulmonary vein with the inspired air, and by the act of expiration is purified from fuliginous vapours, when having become the fit recipient of the vital spirit, it is at length attracted by the diastole." Still very great credit is due to the man who first declared that " the crimson colour is imparted to the spirituous blood by the lungs, not the heart."

Servetus was, however, ignorant of the force by which the blood is impelled into the arteries, and the contractile functions of the heart were unknown. The ventricle was believed to dilate from some undiscovered cause, and thus to suck in the purified " spiritus vitalis." But Servetus's explanation, whatever it was worth, occurred in a theological work, the issue of which led to the author's death at Calvin's persecuting hands, and the work remained unknown—for Calvin carefully burnt every copy possible — until 1694, when Sir Henry Wotton disinterred it.

Realdus Columbus, the associate of Dr. Caius at Padua, had in 1559 published a treatise containing some advanced views, showing that the blood once having entered the right ventricle from the vena cava, cannot return in consequence of the opposition of the tricuspid valves, and he further perceived the effect of the pulmonary valves; but he still held the idea that the blood had to be converted in the lungs into a kind of spirit, and looked upon the liver as the fountain-head of the blood. Finally, he denied the muscular structure of the heart.

Cæsalpinus added to this some more complete idea of the greater circulation, but he knew nothing of the valves in the veins, and held to the belief that there were two kinds of blood, one for the growth, another for the nourishment of the body. He imagined that it was only during sleep that the veins become distended while the pulsations of the arteries become moderated. He had no idea of the connection between the emptying of the arteries and the filling of the veins, nor of the heart being the cause of the blood's movement.

Fabricius, Harvey's teacher of anatomy, had made such a distinct step in advance in discovering the valves of the veins and the effect they must have, that it is quite astonishing that he should not have proceeded farther. But the fact is, that without the microscope as developed in after years,* it was impossible to solve a multitude of questions satisfactorily, and we may rather marvel that Harvey was able to achieve so much with the means at his disposal. The principal means he employed to this end was undoubtedly the vivisection of animals.

Chapter i. of his celebrated treatise on the Motion of the Heart and the Blood (Frankfort, 1628) begins emphatically, "When I first gave my mind to vivisections, as a means of discovering the motions and uses of the heart, and sought to discover these from actual inspection, and not from the writings of others, I found the task so truly arduous, so full of difficulties, that I was almost tempted to think, with Fracastorius, that the motion of the heart was only to be comprehended by God.†

"At length, and by using greater and daily diligence, having frequent recourse to vivisections, employing a variety of animals for the purpose, . . . I thought . . . that I had discovered what I so much desired, with the motion and the use of the heart and arteries. . . .

"These views, as usual, pleased some more, others less; some chid and calumniated me, and laid it to me as a crime that I had dared to depart from the precepts and opinions of all anatomists. . . . At length, yielding

---

* Malpighi first saw the blood circulating. In 1661 he records his having seen the circulation of the blood in the frog's lungs. Later he saw it also in the frog's mesentery.

† Dr. Willis's Translation of Harvey's Works. Sydenham Soc. 1847.

to the requests of my friends, that all might be made
participators in my labours, and partly moved by the
envy of others, who, receiving my views with uncan-
did minds and understanding them indifferently, have
essayed to traduce me publicly, I have been moved to
commit these things to the press. . . . Finally, if any
use or benefit to this department of the republic of
letters should accrue from my labours, it will perhaps
be allowed that I have not lived idly, and, as the old
man in the comedy says :—

> ' For never yet hath any one attained
>   To such perfection, but that time, and place,
>   And use, have brought addition to his knowledge ;
>   Or made correction, or admonished him,
>   That he was ignorant of much which he
>   Had thought he knew ; or led him to reject
>   What he had once esteemed of highest price.'

" So will it, perchance, be found with reference to the
heart at this time; or others, at least, starting from
hence, the way pointed out to them, advancing under
the guidance of a happier genius, may make occasion
to proceed more fortunately, and to inquire more
accurately."

In the second chapter, after a vivid description of
the behaviour of the heart, he thus declares its muscular nature. "The motion of the heart consists in a
certain universal tension—both contraction in the line
of its fibres, and constriction in every sense. It becomes erect, hard, and of diminished size during its

action; the motion is plainly of the same nature as
that of the muscles when they contract in the line of
their sinews and fibres ; for the muscles, when in action,
acquire vigour and tenseness, and from soft become
hard, prominent, and thickened: in the same manner
the heart." . . .

"These things, therefore, happen together or at the
same instant: the tension of the heart, the pulse of its
apex, which is felt externally by its striking against
the chest, the thickening of its parietes, and the forcible
expulsion of the blood it contains by the constriction
of its ventricles."

In further chapters he establishes separately, and in
a masterly manner, the facts that the pulse in the
arteries depends on the contraction of the ventricles ;
that when the left ventricle ceases to contract, the pulse
in the arteries also ceases; that the two auricles contract
together, and also the two ventricles together, but the
ventricles following the auricles in a certain rhythm;
that the heart accomplishes a transfusion of the blood
from the veins to the arteries ; and that the blood sent
into the lungs from the right ventricle passes through
the porous structure of the lungs and back to the left
ventricle.

In his eighth chapter, Harvey feels himself to be
bringing forward considerations of so novel a character,
that "I tremble," he says, "lest I have mankind at
large for my enemies, so much doth wont and custom,
that become as another nature, and doctrine once sown

and that hath struck deep root, and respect for antiquity influence all men : *still the die is cast, and my trust is in my love of truth, and the candour that inheres in cultivated minds.*" He found it impossible to account for the constant influx of blood into the arteries, and the return of blood to the heart, unless there was "a motion, as it were, in a circle." And he shows by calculations of the quantity passing through the heart in an hour, that it is much more than the whole body contains, and that there is no way except by communications taking place from arteries to veins in every part of the body. Finally, he clearly shows how the valves in the veins promote the return of blood to the heart.

Throughout the whole of this treatise considerations from comparative anatomy, from the phenomena of human diseases, and from natural philosophy, are thickly interspersed, and imagery of the most suggestive character is called into requisition; the whole forming a treatise that every scientific man might well read, and that no doctor should consider himself fully educated without having attentively perused. In a subsequent letter to John Riolan the younger, Professor of Anatomy in the University of Paris, Harvey lays down—in opposition to those who repudiate the circulation because they cannot see the efficient nor final cause of it, and who exclaim, *Cui bono ?*—the fundamental scientific axiom, " Our first duty is to inquire whether the thing be or not, before asking wherefore it is." Again, "He who truly desires to be informed of the question in hand, and whether the facts alleged be sensible, visible, or not, must be held bound, either to look for himself, or to take on trust the conclusions to which they have come who have looked; and indeed there is no higher method of attaining to assurance and certainty."

Everything that Harvey wrote shows him to have been pre-eminently an example of the scientific mind, that which submits everything to the test of experiment and observation. Anatomy he professed to learn and teach, not from books, but from dissections, not from the positions of philosophers, but from the fabric of Nature. In the introduction to his Treatise on Generation he praises the "more excellent way" of those "who, following the traces of nature with their own eyes, pursued her through devious but most assured ways till they reached her in the citadel of truth. And truly in such pursuits," he goes on, "it is sweet not merely to toil, but even to grow weary, when the pains of discovering are amply compensated by the pleasures of discovery. Eager for novelty, we are wont to travel far into unknown countries, that with our own eyes we may witness what we have heard reported as having been seen by others, where, however, we for the most part find that the presence lessens the repute. It were disgraceful, therefore, with this most spacious and admirable realm of nature before us, and where the reward ever exceeds the promise, did we take the reports of others upon trust, and go on coining crude problems out of these, and on them hanging knotty and captious and petty disputations. Nature is herself to be addressed; the paths she shows us are to be boldly trodden; for thus, and whilst we consult our proper senses, from inferior advancing to superior levels, shall we penetrate at length into the heart of her mystery."

True and scientific as the Treatise on the Heart and the Circulation was, or rather because it was so true and scientific, its publication gave a decided and severe check to Harvey's professional prosperity. It was believed by the vulgar, says Aubrey, that he was crack-brained. Writing many years after the publication, Aubrey says that though he was allowed to be an excellent anatomist, nobody admired his therapeutic methods. It was said by practitioners that they could not tell by his prescriptions what he aimed at. Yet he continued well in favour with the court, and with numerous persons of distinction. Having become Physician Extraordinary to James I. in 1618 or earlier, he was in 1623 promised the reversion of the office of Physician in Ordinary when a vacancy should occur. But his accession to this post only took place in 1630 under Charles I.*

---

* Harvey's personal history is comparatively little concerned with the controversy which arose in establishing the truth of his discovery. His lectures and demonstrations at the College of Physicians were so convincing that he met with but slight opposition from capable critics in England. Continental professors, however, were slower to accept his teaching. "The Circulation of the Blood," he says in his first answer

Harvey became Treasurer of the College of Physicians in 1628, but resigned this office and also procured the appointment of a deputy at St. Bartholomew's Hospital in 1630, when he was commanded by the King to attend the young Duke of Lennox in his travels on the Continent. Having returned from this expedition, in 1632 he was sworn in Physician in Ordinary for his Majesty's household, and in 1639 we find a letter in the Lord Steward's office, giving orders for settling a diet of three dishes of meat a meal with all incidents thereunto belonging upon Dr. Harvey. But later on, in 1640, the King when at York makes another arrangement, devoting £200 a year to Dr. Harvey, the three dishes of meat probably not having been readily forthcoming just then. In 1632–3 a deputy had again to be appointed at St. Bartholomew's; in 1636 he was required to accompany the Earl of Arundel on his embassy to the Emperor of Germany. This gave him an opportunity of personally explaining the circulation to various eminent physicians in the principal German cities. On one of these occasions, at Nuremberg, we find it recorded that Harvey gave a public demonstration of the circulation, which satisfied

---

to Riolan in 1649, "has now been before the world for many years, illustrated by proofs cognizable to the senses, and confirmed by numerous experiments; but no one has yet attempted opposition to it on the ground of ocular testimony. Empty assertions, baseless arguments, captious cavillings, and contumelious epithets are all that have been levelled against the doctrine and its author." We need not, therefore, follow here the history of the final and full triumph of Harvey's views on the Continent.

all except Caspar Hofmann.* Returning to England, Harvey accompanied Charles I. in his expeditions, such as that to Scotland in 1639; and we may remark that, being in such close proximity to the royal person, he contrived very skilfully not to become involved in court intrigues, his best protection being his devotion to his medical and physiological investigations.† Even when war had broken out, Harvey became in no way obnoxious to the Parliament, for he tells us himself that he attended the King not only with the consent but by the desire of Parliament. In this way Harvey was present on the very field at the battle of Edgehill.

"During the fight," says Aubrey, "the Prince and

* That Harvey's scientific ardour was in full operation during this journey we also learn from a remark of Hollar the artist, who accompanied the ambassador : " He would still be making of excursions into the wood, making observations of strange trees, plants, earths, &c., and sometimes like to be lost ; so that my lord ambassador would be really angry with him, for there was not only danger of wild beasts, but of thieves."

In a letter written on this journey, Harvey says : "By the way we could scarce see a dog, crow, kite, raven, or any bird, or anything to anatomize ; only some few miserable people, the reliques of the war and the plague, whom famine had made anatomies before I came."

† There is every reason to believe that by this course of conduct Harvey lost nothing of the King's favour and regard. Harvey records that on several occasions the King had exhibited to him the beating heart of the chick in the shell. We learn that he placed at Harvey's disposal several does for his experiments, and was present on various occasions at his dissections. Though it is not definitely recorded, Harvey appears to have accompanied Charles on at least one of his journeys to Scotland, and to have visited the Bass Rock. In his work on Generation he incidentally describes the seabirds which he found so abundant there.

Duke of York were committed to his care. He told me that he withdrew with them under a hedge, and took out of his pocket a book and read. But he had not read very long before a bullet of a great gun grazed on the ground near him, which made him remove his station." We cannot but admire the coolness and serenity of mind which could thus occupy itself with reading in the midst of carnage, having evidently no sort of belief in, or vocation for, the employment of force in the arbitrament between opposing opinions. Accompanying Charles to Oxford, he found congenial society, and was incorporated Doctor of Medicine on the 7th December, 1642. " I first saw him at Oxford," says Aubrey, " 1642, after Edgehill fight; but was then too young to be acquainted with so great a doctor. I remember he came several times to our college (Trinity) to George Bathurst, B.D., who had a hen to hatch eggs in his chamber, which they opened daily to see the progress and way of generation."

Thus we see Harvey continuing engaged in that study of the mysteries of reproduction and development to which he devoted so many years and so many toils. He must have commenced his studies on this subject at least early in Charles's reign.

In 1645, while the King and his physician still remained at Oxford, Sir Nathaniel Brent having quitted Merton College, of which he was Warden, and taken the Covenant, Harvey was appointed Warden in his place by virtue of a royal mandate. He had indeed lost more than his time in following the royal fortunes, and deserved any reward the King could bestow upon him. At the close of the sixty-eighth section of his treatise on Generation Harvey says, " Let gentle minds forgive me if, recalling the irreparable injuries I have suffered, I here give vent to a sigh. This is the cause of my sorrow: whilst in attendance on his Majesty during our late troubles and more than civil wars, not only with the permission but by the command of the Parliament, certain rapacious hands stripped not only my house of all its furniture, but what is subject of far greater regret with me, my enemies abstracted from my museum the fruits of many years of toil. Whence it has come to pass that many observations, particularly on the generation of insects, have perished, with detriment, I venture to say, to the republic of letters." *

The Wardenship of Merton was not long Dr. Harvey's, for when Oxford surrendered to the Parliamentary forces in July 1646, he quitted the university and returned to London, and Sir Nathaniel Brent was reinstated in his former position. Nothing has been ascertained of the reason for Harvey's cessation of personal attendance on the King at this period, but it is certain that he took

* It is in reference to this that Cowley says :—

"O cursed war ! who can forgive thee this ?
Houses and towns may rise again,
And ten times easier 'tis
To rebuild Paul's than any work of his."

refuge in the homes of his brothers, each of whom, whether in the City, at Lambeth, at Roehampton, or at Combe, kept special apartments reserved for him. It is most pleasing, indeed, to note the great brotherly affection existing in this family. The earliest of them to die, Thomas Harvey, in 1622, has the following inscription on his monumental tablet. " As in a Sheaf of Arrows. *Vis unita fortior.* The Band of Love the Uniter of Brethren." Thus, leaving his financial concerns in charge of his brother Eliab, William devoted himself, at the age of sixty-eight, more fully to his researches on Generation, which his friend Dr. Ent extracted from him at Christmas 1650.

Dr. Ent, addressing the President and Fellows of the College of Physicians, writes an introduction to this work, in which he gives us a pleasing view of Harvey in his retirement. He says: " Harassed with anxious, and in the end not much availing cares, about Christmas last, I sought to rid my spirit of the cloud which oppressed it by a visit to that great man, the chief honour and ornament of our college, Dr. William Harvey, then dwelling not far from the city. I found him, Democritus like, busy with the study of natural things, his countenance cheerful, his mind serene, embracing all within its sphere. I forthwith saluted him, and asked if all were well with him. ' How can it,' said he, ' while the Commonwealth is full of distractions, and I myself am still in the open sea ? And truly,' he continued, ' did I not find solace in my studies, and a balm for my spirit in the memory of my observations of former years, I should feel little desire for longer life. But so it has been, that this life of obscurity, this vacation from public business, which causes tedium and disgust to so many, has proved a sovereign remedy to me.' " An extended conversation is recorded, in which Harvey discourses in his wisest vein on the value of the interrogation of nature in every possible way. Dr. Ent informed him that the learned world were eagerly looking for his further experiments. Harvey rejoined, " You know full well what a storm my former lucubrations raised. Much better is it oftentimes to grow wise at home and in private, than by publishing what you have amassed with infinite labour, to stir up tempests that may rob you of peace and quiet for the rest of your days." He at last produced the treatise on generation of animals, and Dr. Ent urging him to publish it both in consideration of his own fame, and the public benefit, and offering to see it through the press, the author consented to its publication at once or at some future time. Dr. Ent was exultant, feeling, like another Jason, laden with the golden fleece. " Our Harvey," he says, " rather seems as though discovery were natural to him, a thing of ease and of course, a matter of ordinary business ; though he may nevertheless have expended infinite labour and study on his works. And we have evidence of his singular candour in this, that he never hostilely attacks any previous writer, but ever courteously sets down and comments upon the opinions of each ; and indeed he is wont to say, that it is argument of an indifferent cause when it is contended for with violence and distemper, and that truth scarce wants an advocate."

This great work, published in 1651, begins by describing the hen's egg and its development, the doctrine being enunciated that all animals as well as plants are produced from ova.   Incidentally, as well as subsequently, observations of great merit and value on reproduction in all kinds of animals are given, and it is clearly shown that instead of containing, from the first, excessively minute but complete animals, eggs at first include extremely simple structures, which by successive and gradual changes come to be like the adults from which they have sprung,   It is true that Harvey, with Aristotle, believed that the germs of lower animals could arise out of non-living matter ; but it is only in the most recent days that the most elaborate microscopical investigations seem finally to have disposed of this view.   The doctrine that the simply constructed germ grows by feeding on non-living matter, converting it into living matter, and gradually transforming it into the form characterising the parent, was a great innovation in Harvey's age, and it hung fire till Caspar Wolff, in 1759, securely established it. But this has remained till the present century to be made fruitful.

Throughout Harvey's treatise it is evident how greatly the lack of powers such as those of the microscope crippled the entire investigation, although it is truly wonderful how much was accomplished without its aid. Incidental remarks show the acute mind everywhere tending towards sound procedure, as in tying the main artery of a tumour he wished to destroy ; arriving on the brink of a discovery even when its full perception did not come, as when in regard to the lungs he says, " Air is given neither for the cooling nor the nutrition of animals," contrary to the prevailing notion. But the absence of chemical knowledge in that age prevented his going farther.

His published works only represent a portion of Harvey's life-work. We find allusions to his " Medical Observations " and " Medical Anatomy," which, if written, were probably destroyed in the College of Physicians at the Great Fire. In one place Harvey states that in his medical anatomy he meant, " from the many dissections he had made of the bodies of persons worn out by serious and strange affections, to relate how and in what way the internal organs were changed in their situation, size, structure, figure, consistency, and other sensible qualities, from their natural forms and appearances, such as they are usually described by anatomists, and in what various and remarkable ways they were affected. For even as the dissection of healthy and well-constituted bodies contributes essentially to the advancement of philosophy and sound physiology, so does the inspection of diseased and cachectic subjects powerfully assist philosophical pathology." Thus it appears that, had we possessed Harvey's pathological observations, he would also have merited the title of founder of pathology.

About the time of the publication of the Treatise on Generation, Harvey's work on the Heart and Circulation was gaining continued and widespread adhesion on the Continent. In Italy, Trullius, a Roman professor; in France, John Pecquet of Dieppe; in Leyden, Thomas Bartholin, were occupied in promulgating Harvey's views. A notable convert was Plempius of Louvain, who, having given himself up to the refutation of Harvey, found himself compelled to retract when he himself made some experiments on living dogs.

Harvey was constantly solicitous for the welfare of the College of Physicians, before which he continued to deliver the Lumleian Lectures up to 1656. At an extraordinary meeting held on 4th July, 1651, Dr. Prujean, the President, read to the Fellows the following anonymous proposal : " If I can procure one that will build us a library, and a repository for simples and rarities, such a one as shall be suitable and honourable to the college, will you assent to have it done or no ? " The offer was of course unanimously and gratefully accepted, but it does not appear at what period it transpired that Harvey was the munificent donor. However, on 22d December, 1652, the college decreed a statue to him, which was executed in his doctor's cap and gown, inscribed " Viro monumentis suis immortali."

It was not, however, till the 2d of February, 1653-4, that the new building was opened, consisting, as Aubrey tells us, of a noble building of Roman architecture (of rustic work with Corinthian pilasters), comprising a great parlour, a kind of convocation-room for the Fellows to meet in below, and a library above. Harvey was present on the opening occasion, having provided a handsome entertainment, and formally handed over the title-deeds and entire interest in the building in a speech of the utmost benevolence and goodwill. He had contributed not merely the building, but also a considerable library, and many surgical instruments and objects of interest to the museum.

On the 30th September, 1654, Harvey was elected in his absence to the presidency of the college, which, however, he declined on the next day, owing to his age and growing infirmities, and recommending the continuance in office of Dr. Prujean, who nominated him as one of the council, which office he did not refuse. He continued to lecture, although his strength was diminished by severe attacks of gout, but in July 1656 he resigned his lectureship. In taking leave of the college, at a grand banquet which he gave, he presented it with his patrimonial estate at Burmarsh in Kent. One special provision settled a salary for a librarian, and another established what has since been known as the Harveian Oration, delivered yearly in commemoration of benefactors to the college, and now extended to those who have added to medical science during the year.

The long and truly fortunate career of Harvey—for fortunate he must be deemed, who, like Darwin, having enunciated an epoch-making discovery, lived to see it inculcated as a canon—was now drawing to a close. In several of his later letters he expresses his feelings of infirmity. Writing in 1655 to Dr. Horst, at Hesse-Darmstadt, he speaks of "advanced age, which unfits us for the investigation of novel subtleties, and the mind which inclines to repose after the fatigues of lengthened labours." Later, on the 24th April, 1657, writing to Dr. Vlackveld, at Harlem, he says: "It is in vain that you apply the spur to urge me, at my present age—not mature merely, but declining—to gird myself for any new investigation. For I now consider myself entitled to my discharge from duty."

Harvey died on the 3d of June, 1657, in the eightieth year of his age, and the Fellows of his college followed his remains far out of the city towards Hempstead, in Essex, where his brother Eliab had a vault. His will is a characteristic document. He thus expresses his Christian faith: "I do most humbly render my soul to Him that gave it, and to my blessed Lord and Saviour Christ Jesus." Making his brother Eliab executor and residuary legatee, he bequeaths legacies to all his relations with most affectionate expressions: we do not know the date of his wife's death (she was still living in 1645), but she is here mentioned as "my

dear deceased loving wife." " I give to the College of
Physicians all my books and papers, and my best
Persia long carpet, and my blue satin embroidered
cushion, one pair of brass andirons, with fireshovel and
tongs of brass, for the ornament of the meeting-room
I have erected." It seems very probable that these
books and papers included some much-regretted observations of Harvey's, which were destroyed, with the building which he erected and the statue to his memory,
in the great fire of 1666. He left £10 to his friend
Hobbes of Malmesbury, who describes Harvey as the
only one that he knew who conquered envy and established a new doctrine in his lifetime.

" The private character of this great man," says
Aikin, in his Biographical Memoirs of Medicine in
Great Britain, "appears to have been in every respect
worthy of his public reputation. Cheerful, candid, and
upright, he was not the prey of any mean or ungentle
passion. He was as little disposed by nature to detract
from the merits of others, or make an ostentatious display of his own, as necessitated to use such methods
for advancing his fame. The many antagonists whom
his renown and the novelty of his opinions excited
were, in general, treated by him with modest and tem-
perate language, frequently very different from their
own ; and while he refuted their arguments, he decorated
them with all due praises. He lived on terms of perfect harmony and friendship with his brethren of the
college; and seems to have been very little ambitious

of engrossing a disproportionate share of medical
practice. In extreme old age, pain and sickness were
said to have rendered him somewhat irritable in his
temper. . . . It is certain that the profoundest venera-
tion for the great Cause of all those wonders he was so
well acquainted with appears eminently conspicuous
in every part of his works. He was used to say, that
he never dissected the body of any animal without discovering something which he had not expected or conceived of, and in which he recognised the hand of an
all-wise Creator. To His particular agency, and not to
the operation of general laws, he ascribed all the phenomena of nature. In familiar conversation Harvey was
easy and unassuming, and singularly clear in express-
ing his ideas. His mind was furnished with an ample
store of knowledge, not only in matters connected with
his profession, but in most of the objects of liberal
inquiry, especially in ancient and modern history, and
the science of politics. He took great delight in reading the ancient poets, Virgil in particular, with whose
divine productions he is said to have been sometimes
so transported as to throw the book from him with
exclamations of rapture. To complete his character, he
did not want that polish and courtly address which
are necessary to the scholar who would also appear as
a gentleman."

According to Aubrey, who knew him well, Harvey
was not tall, but of the lowest stature; round-faced,
olivaster in complexion, with little round eyes, very

black and full of spirit, his hair black as a raven,
but quite white twenty years before he died. His
portrait in the College of Physicians corresponds with
this account, indicating a nervous, bilious temperament,
and showing a compact, square, wide forehead. The
general expression is highly intellectual, contemplative,
and manly.

Harvey has the rare distinction of standing at the
head of three departments of science in England—comparative anatomy, physiology, and medicine. When
these scarcely existed, he evolved them into living form
from chaos. The extent of his achievements must be
gauged by the extent of the superstructure built upon
his foundations. He laid the foundations broad and
firm, and practised the true method of science. Notwithstanding Harvey's infirmities, his mind in old
age was characterised by an abiding youthfulness and
desire to learn, so that Aubrey found him studying
Oughtred's "Clavis Mathematica," and working problems not long before he died. He was equally pleased
to communicate his knowledge to others, and, as Aubrey
relates, "to instruct any that were modest and re-
spectful to him. In order to my journey (I was at
that time bound for Italy), he dictated to me what
to see, what company to keep, what books to read,
how to manage my studies—in short, he bid me go
to the fountain-head and read Aristotle, Cicero, Avi-
cenna." He was always very contemplative, and was
wont to frequent the leads of Cockaine House,

which his brother Eliab had bought, having there his several stations in regard to the sun and the wind, for the indulgence of his fancy. At the house at Combe, in Surrey, he had caves made in the ground, in which he delighted in the summer-time to meditate. He also loved darkness, as he could then best contemplate. The activity of his mind would often deprive him of sleep, when he would rise and walk about in his shirt, until he was cooled and could gain sleep. Similarly he treated his attacks of gout; he would sit with his legs bare, even in frost, on the leads of Cockaine House, and put them into a pail of water until he was almost dead with cold, and thus he found his attacks could be moderated.

His great works were, according to the custom of the age, written in Latin; and Dr. Willis, who has translated all of them into English, describes his Latin as generally easy, often elegant, and not unfrequently copious and imaginative—he never seems to feel in the least fettered by the language he is using.

The College of Physicians, says Dr. Munk, possesses some interesting memorials of Harvey, two of which may be mentioned. One the whalebone probe or rod, tipped with silver, with which he demonstrated the parts in his Lumleian Lectures at the college. The other, consisting of six tables of wood, upon which are spread the different blood-vessels and nerves of the human body, carefully dissected out, probably prepared by Harvey himself, and presumed to have been used by him in his lectures. They were presented to the college by the Earl of Winchelsea, one of whose ancestors, the Lord-Chancellor Nottingham, had married the niece of Harvey.

CHAPTER III.

THOMAS SYDENHAM, THE BRITISH HIPPOCRATES.

IN the front rank of practical physicians in England stands THOMAS SYDENHAM, descended from an ancient Somersetshire family, one branch of which migrated into Dorsetshire in the reign of Henry VIII., and settled at Winford Eagle. Here he was born in 1624. We know nothing of his early years till we find him entered at Magdalen Hall, Oxford, in 1642. His studies were interrupted by Charles I.'s residence there, and it is very probable that he took arms on the side of the Parliament, while it is certain that his brothers did so—one of them, William Sydenham, having been a well-known Parliamentarian commissioner, and Governor of the Isle of Wight. His mother, too, was in some way, of which we have no account, "killed in the civil wars" in 1644, so that there is sufficient reason why Thomas Sydenham should have withdrawn from Oxford at this time. Sir Richard Blackmore indeed describes him as a disbanded officer, and this appears possible from what Sydenham himself states.

In his letter dedicatory to Dr. John Mapletoft of

the third edition of his "Medical Observations," Sydenham says: "It is now thirty years since I had the
good fortune to fall in with the learned and ingenu-
ous Master Thomas Coxe, Doctor. . . . I myself was
on my way to London, with the intention of going
thence to Oxford, the breaking out of the war having
kept me away for some years. With his well-known
kindness and condescension, Dr. Coxe asked me what
pursuit I was prepared to make my profession. . . .
Upon this point my mind was unfixed, whilst I had
not so much as dreamed of medicine. Stimulated,
however, by the recommendation and encouragement of
so high an authority, I prepared myself seriously for
that pursuit. Hence all the little merit that my works
may have earned in the eyes of the public is to be
thankfully referred to him who was the patron and
promoter of my first endeavours."

Dr. Lettsom in 1801 communicated to the *Gentleman's Magazine* a MS. anecdote which has since
been found to be derived from "The Vindicatory
Schedule," by Dr. Andrew Brown, published two years
after Sydenham's death. "Dr. Thos. Sydenham was
an actor in the late civil war, and discharged the office
of captain. He being in his lodgings in London, and
going to bed at night with his clothes loosed, a mad
drunken fellow, a soldier, likewise in the same lodging,
entered his room, with one hand gripping him by the
breast of his shirt, with the other discharged a loaded
pistol into his bosom ; yet, oh strange ! without any hurt

to him." The story then goes on to relate how the
bullet happened to be discharged in the line of all the
bones of the palm of the hand edgeways, so that it lost
its force and was spent without doing any harm to
Sydenham.

When Oxford surrendered to the Parliament, Sydenham returned to Magdalen Hall, and was soon afterwards elected a fellow of All Souls' in place of an
expelled Royalist. The degree of M.B. he took in 1648,
without taking a degree in arts; and he appears to
have resided at Oxford for some years, with possibly an
interval spent at the Montpellier School of Medicine.
Soon after taking his degree he began to suffer from
gout and symptoms of stone, to which he was a martyr
more or less for the rest of his life.

We do not know in what year Sydenham finally
quitted Oxford and went to London. He gives an
account of the epidemics of 1661 in London, where he
must then have been settled. In 1663 he became a
licentiate of the College of Physicians, but could not
proceed further without a doctor's degree, which he did
not take till comparatively late in life, in 1676.

In 1666 appeared Sydenham's first work, the first
edition of the "Method of Curing Fevers," dealing with
continued and intermittent fevers, and with smallpox.

This first edition was dedicated to Robert Boyle,
whom Sydenham describes as "truly and wholly
noble," and to whom he ascribes transcendent parts,
such as to raise him to the level of the most famous

names of foregone ages. He acknowledges many and
great favours conferred upon him by his friend; and
he states soberly that it was on Boyle's persuasion and
recommendation that he undertook to write the book,
and by his experience that some portions of it had
been tested. Boyle occasionally accompanied Sydenham in his visits to the sick. The physician hopes his
book will not find less favour for being "neither vast
in bulk, nor stuffed out with the spoils of former
authors." "I have no wish to disturb their ashes," he
remarks.

The preface to the first edition begins thus: "Who-
ever takes up medicine should seriously consider the
following points: firstly, that he must one day render to the Supreme Judge an account of the lives of
those sick men who have been intrusted to his care.
Secondly, that such skill and science as, by the blessing of God, he has attained, are to be specially directed
towards the honour of his Maker and the welfare of his
fellow-creatures, since it is a base thing for the great
gifts of heaven to become the servants of avarice or
ambition. Thirdly, he must remember that it is no
mean ignoble animal that he deals with. We may ascertain the worth of the human race, since for its sake
God's only-begotten Son became man, and thereby
ennobled the nature that He took upon Him. Lastly,
he must remember that he himself hath no exemption
from the common lot, but that he is bound by the same
laws of mortality, and liable to the same ailments and

afflictions with his fellows. For these and like reasons let him strive to render aid to the distressed with the greater care, with the kindlier spirit, and with the stronger fellow-feeling."

The candid and philosophic temperament of the man is also well exemplified in the conclusion of the same preface. He foresees that " even where my practice has been tried, and its results been recognised, it will be asserted that my statements are anything but new, and that the world has long known them. I have, notwithstanding, never allowed myself to be deterred from communicating the following pages to those of my fellow-creatures who unite the love of truth with the love of their kind. It is my temper and disposition to be careless both of the sayings and the doings of the over-proud and the over-critical. To the wise, however, and the honest, I wish to say this much :—I have in no wise distorted either fact or experiment ; I told the truth, the whole truth, and nothing but the truth. . . . In the meanwhile I ask the pardon, and submit to the arguments, of better judges than myself, for all errors of theory. Perhaps I may myself hereafter on many points change my mind of my own accord. As I have no lack of charity for the errors of others, I have no love of obstinately persisting in my own."

At the outset of his treatise he asserts that a disease is an effort of nature which strives with might and main to restore the health of the patient by the elimination of the morbific matter. Yet he is so far in accord with

modern discovery of bacterial germs, that he refers the
specific differences between fevers to some unknown
constitution of the atmosphere. His wisdom is conspicuous when he says he prefers nothing, on the out-
break of a new fever, to a little delay, and diligently
observes the character and cause of the disease, and
what kinds of treatment do good or harm. He discerns
thoroughly that the scientific working out of the characteristics and phenomena of each disease must be
accomplished before it can be asserted that any good
work worthy of mention has been got through. It would
be difficult to exhibit a more modest and a more truly
philosophical spirit than that shown in the following
lines at the close of his second chapter : " One thing
most especially do I aim at. It is my wish to state
how things have gone lately ; how they have been in
this the city which we live in. The observations of
some years form my groundwork. It is thus that I
would add my mite, such as it is, towards the foundation of a work that, in my humble judgment, shall be
beneficial to the human race. Posterity will complete
it, since to them it shall be given to take the full
view of the whole cycle of epidemics in their mutual
sequences for years yet to come."

A signal instance of his philosophic moderation is
given in the following extract: " For my own part, I
am not ambitious of the name of a philosopher, and
those who think themselves so, may perhaps consider
me blameable on the score of my not having attempted

to pierce into those penetralia. Now, writers like these I would just recommend, before they blame others, to try their hand upon some common phenomena of nature that meet us at every turn. For instance, I would fain know why a horse attains its prime at seven, and a man at one-and-twenty years ? Why, in the vegetable kingdom, some plants blow in May and others in June ? There are numberless questions of this sort. Hence, if many men of consummate wisdom are not ashamed to proclaim their ignorance in these matters, I cannot see why I am to be called in question for doing the same. Etiology is a difficult, and, perhaps, an inexplicable affair; and I choose to keep my hands clear of it. *I am convinced, however, that Nature here, as elsewhere, moves in a regular and orderly manner.*"

In how wise and firm a tone does Sydenham denounce and demolish the quacks and patent medicine vendors ! He considers that any man who can, by any sure line of treatment, or by the application of any specific remedy, control the course of diseases or cut them short, is bound by every possible bond to reveal to the world in general so great a blessing to his race. If he withheld it, he pronounced him a bad citizen and an unwise man; for no good citizen would monopolise for himself a general benefit for his kind, and no wise man would divest himself of the blessing he might reasonably expect from his Maker in contributing to the welfare of the world.

Sydenham stands out as a great advocate and champion of Peruvian bark, which, in its modern form of quinine, has justified all that he claimed for it. He is also the founder of the "expectant" treatment. "My chief care," he says, "in the midst of so much darkness and ignorance, is to wait a little, and proceed very slowly, especially in the use of powerful remedies, in the meantime observing its nature and procedure, and by what means the patient was relieved or injured."

The new treatise at once attracted attention, and was reviewed in the Philosophical Transactions for 1666. In the same year there appeared a Dutch edition of the Method. The value and the effect of this treatise we can scarcely fully appreciate at the present time, but its pith is well given by Dr. John Brown, author of the "Horæ Subsecivæ." "Besides their broad, accurate, vivid delineations of disease—portraits drawn to the life, and by a great master—and their wise, simple, rational rules for treatment, active and negative, general and specific—there are two great principles continually referred to as supreme in the art of medicine. The first is that nature cures diseases; that there is a recuperative and curative power, the *vis medicatrix*, in every living organism, implanted in it by the Almighty, and that it is by careful reverential scrutiny of this law of restoration that all our attempts at cure are to be guided; that we are its ministers and interpreters, and neither more nor less; and the second, that symptoms are the language of a suffering and disordered and endangered body, which it is the duty of the physician

to listen to, and as far as he can to explain and satisfy,
and that, like all other languages, it must be studied.
This is what he calls the natural history of diseases.
. . . What Locke did for the science of mind, what
Harvey and Newton did for the sciences of organic and
inorganic matter, Sydenham did for the art of healing
and of keeping men whole : he made it in the main
observational ; he founded it upon what he himself
calls downright matter of fact, and did this not by
unfolding a system of doctrines or raising up a scaffold-
ing of theory, but by pointing to a road, by exhibiting
a method—and moreover teaching this by example, not
less than by precept—walking in the road, not acting
merely as a finger-post, and showing himself to be
throughout a true artsman and master of his tools.
The value he puts upon sheer, steady, honest observation, as the one initial act and process of all true science
of nature, is most remarkable ; and he gives himself, in
his descriptions of disease in general and of particular
cases, proofs quite exquisite of his own powers of persevering, minute, truthful scrutiny."

In 1668 a second edition of the Method was published,
with additions, especially a chapter on the Plague,
and prefaced by a eulogistic address in Latin verse,
extending to fifty-four lines, by the illustrious Locke.
In 1676 appeared the third edition of the Method,
so much enlarged that it is better regarded as the first
edition of the "Medical Observations." In the same
year Sydenham proceeded to the degree of Doctor of

Medicine, not at Oxford, but at Cambridge, this choice being probably due to the fact that his son had entered at Pembroke College, Cambridge, two years before.

From the preface to his treatise on gout and dropsy, published in 1683, we find that Sydenham was compelled to lay aside his project of a complete book on chronic diseases by the extreme attacks of gout which his labours brought on. "Whenever I returned to my studies," he says, "my gout returned to me." A few years before, in 1677, he had been prevented from practising by a severe attack of gout, and he was compelled to spend another three months in the country to restore his health. He continued his labours, however, it is to be believed, beyond his strength, and several editions of his works, with fresh observations, were issued in the later years of his life. He died at his house in Pall Mall on the 29th of December, 1689, aged sixty-five, being buried at St. James's, Westminster. The truly appropriate description, "Medicus in omne aevum nobilis," was given of him by the College of Physicians in 1810, when a mural tablet was raised to his memory near his place of burial.

Sydenham's will shows that he had three sons—William, Henry, and James—the eldest of whom received entailed estates in Hertfordshire and Leicestershire. He bequeathed £30 for the professional education of his nephew James, afterwards Sir James Thornhill, Hogarth's father-in-law. Sydenham's executor was Mr. Malthus, an apothecary of Pall Mall (great-grandfather of Professor Malthus), whom he enjoins to bury him with a careful abstinence from all ostentatious funeral pomp.

It is perhaps not necessary to regret so acutely the lack of biographical details regarding Dr. Sydenham, as many have done, for we think that his character stands out clearly in his writings.   In his letter to Dr. Mapletoft, already referred to, he says :—

" After a few years spent in the arena of the university, I returned to London for the practice of medicine. The more I observed the facts of this science with an attentive eye, and the more I studied them with due and proper diligence, the more I became confirmed in the opinion which I have held up to the present hour, viz., *that the art of medicine was to be properly learnt only from its practice and its exercise ;* and that, in all probability, he would be the best skilled in the detection of the true and genuine indications of treatment who had the most diligently and the most accurately attended to the natural phenomena of disease."

The same preface contains Sydenham's opinion of a great contemporary and valued friend of his.   "You know also how thoroughly an intimate and common friend, and one who has closely and exhaustively examined the question, agrees with me as to the method I am speaking of—a man who, in the acuteness of his intellect, in the steadiness of his judgment, in the simplicity (and by *simplicity* I mean *excellence*) of his manners, has amongst the present generation few equals and no superiors. This praise I may confidently attach to the name of John Locke." Dugald Stewart, commenting on this, says: " The merit of the Method therefore may be presumed to have belonged in part to Mr. Locke." There is no reason, however, in the co-operation of these great minds, for detracting from the praise of either.

Sydenham's idea of a satisfactory method of curing was a line of practice based upon a sufficient number of experiments. His business was, he says, to support his own observations, not to discuss the opinions of others. The facts would speak for themselves, and would alone show whether he acted with truth and honesty, or, like a profligate and immoral man, was to be a murderer even when in his grave. In the preface to the third edition he says, " The breath of life would have been to me a vain gift, unless I contributed my mite to the treasury of physic." He considered that medicine was to be advanced in two main ways—by a history of diseases, by descriptions at once graphic and natural, and by formulating a praxis or method of treating them. The most modern thought could pro-duce no sounder principle for describing disease than the following: "In writing the history of a disease, every philosophical hypothesis whatsoever that has previously occupied the mind of the author should lie in abeyance. This being done, the clear and natural phenomena of the disease should be noted—these and these only. These should be noted accurately and in all their minuteness." He wittily remarks that it often happens that the character of the complaint varies with the nature of the remedies, and that symptoms may be referred less to the disease than to the doctor. He traces the lack of accurate descriptions of diseases to an idea that disease was but a confused and disordered effort of nature defending herself in vain, so that men had classed the attempts at a just description with the attempts to wash blackamoors white.

Sydenham conceived the idea, too, of paying some attention to the wishes and tastes of the patient. "A person in a burning fever desires to drink freely of some small liquor; but the rules of art, built upon some hypothesis, having a different design in view, thwart the desire, and instead thereof order a cordial. In the meantime the patient, not being suffered to drink what he wishes, nauseates all kinds of food, but art commands him to eat. Another, after a long illness, begs hard, it may be, for something odd or questionable; here, again, impertinent art thwarts him and threatens him with death. How much more excellent the aphorism of Hippocrates: 'Such food as is most grateful, though not so wholesome, is to be preferred to that which is better, but distasteful.'" He has nothing of the meddlesome practitioner about him. "Indeed, if I may speak my mind freely, I have been long of opinion that I act the part of an honest man and a good physician as often as I refrain entirely from medicines, when, upon visiting the patient, I find him no worse to-day than he was yesterday; whereas, if I attempt to cure the patient by a method of which I am uncertain, he will be endangered both by the experiment I am going to make on him and by the disease itself; nor will he so easily escape two dangers as one."

A fine description of one aspect of hysteria and hypochondria may here be given as an example of his power in the delineation of disease: "The patients believe that they have to suffer all the evils that can befall humanity, all the troubles that the world can supply. They have melancholy forebodings, they brood over trifles, cherishing them in their anxious and unquiet bosoms. Fear, anger, jealousy, suspicion, and the worst passions of the mind arise without cause. Joy, hope, cheerfulness, if they find place at all in their spirits, find it at intervals 'few and far between,' and then take leave quickly. In these, as in the painful feelings, there is no moderation. All is caprice. They love without measure those whom they will soon hate without reason. Now they will do this, now that—ever receding from their purpose. . . . All that they see in their dreams are funerals and the shadows of departed friends."

The great physician has nowhere described his own character more clearly than in the following passage: "In all points of theory where the reader finds me in error, I ask his pardon. In all points of practice I state that I speak nothing but the truth; and that I have propounded nothing except what I have properly

tried.   Verily, I am sure that, when the last day of my
life shall have come upon me, I shall carry in my heart
a willing witness that shall speak, not only to the care
and honesty with which I have laboured for the health
of both rich and poor who have intrusted themselves
to my care, but also to those efforts which I have made
to the best of my power, and with all the energies of
my mind, to give certainty to the treatment of diseases
even after my death, if such may be.   In the first place,
no patient has been treated by me otherwise than I
would myself wish to be treated under the same complaint.   In the second, I have ever held that any accession whatever to the art of healing, even if it went
no further than the cutting of corns or the curing of
toothaches, was of far higher value than all the knowledge of fine points, and all the pomp of subtle specula-
tions—matters which are as useful to physicians in
driving away diseases, as music is to masons in laying
bricks."

The last comparison leads us to note that a vein of
humour runs through Sydenham's works, as when he
quotes

"Tua res agitur paries quum proximus ardet,"

as a reason for his leaving London in the height of the
plague.

In another passage, he is referring to the want of
opportunity of the poor to injure themselves by unsuitable diet in smallpox, owing to the "res augusta

domi." Yet even among the poor, he says, since they
learnt the use of certain cordials, many more have died
than in previous ages less learned but more wise.
"Nowadays every house has its old woman," he says,
" a practitioner in an art she never learnt, to the killing
of mankind."

In one place he grimly remarks, that if a certain
mode of treatment be resorted to, the patient will die
of his own doctor, an end which in that age must have
too frequently resulted, though not specified in the
catalogue of diseases.

Here is a specimen of Sydenham's witty apophthegms :
" A man who finds a treasure lying on the ground before
him, is a fool if he do not stoop and pick it up ; but
he is a greater one who, on the strength of such a single
piece of luck, wastes labour and risks life for the chance
of another."

Again, "The usual pomp of medicine exhibited over
dying patients is like the garlands of a beast at the sacri-
fice." Elsewhere he refers to some persons "to whom
nature has given just wit enough to traduce her with."
We must also refer to Sydenham's humour his answer to
Sir Richard Blackmore, who asked him what books he
should study medicine in : "Read Don Quixote, sir,
which is a very good book : I read it still."

We notice as an instance of Sydenham's kind-hearted-
ness, a case in which he lent a poor man one of his
horses for a several days' journey, believing continuous
horse-exercise to be the best cure for his disease.

Another characteristic touch is the following: "I have always thought that to have published for the benefit of afflicted mortals any certain method of subduing even the slightest disease, was a matter of greater felicity than the riches of a Tantalus or a Croesus." To Dr. Brady he remarks: "To you that undeserved abuse wherewith I am harassed by many, is a vexation and sorrow; whilst, of those who utter it this I may safely say, that if a harmless life, hurting none by word or deed, had been sufficient to protect me from their tongues, they never would have thundered against me. Since, then, it is from no fault of mine that these calumnies have fallen on me, this is my resolution, viz., that I will not afflict myself because other men have done wrong."

Again he says: "My fame is in the hands of others. I have weighed in a nice and scrupulous balance, whether it be better to serve men, or to be praised by them, and I prefer the former. It does more to tranquillise the mind; whereas fame, and the breath of popular applause, is but a bubble, a feather, and a dream. Such wealth as such fame gives, those who have scraped it together, and those who value it highly, are fully free to enjoy, only let them remember that the mechanical arts (and sometimes the meanest of them) bring greater gains, and make richer heirs."

He addressed to Dr. Thomas Short his treatise on Gout and Dropsy, because "although others despised the observations which I previously published, you had no hesitation in attributing to them some utility." . . . "It is my nature to think where others read; to ask less whether the world agrees with me than whether I agree with the truth; and to hold cheap the rumour and applause of the multitude."

We have yet to note a remarkable fragment entitled " Theologia Rationalis, by Dr. Thomas Sydenham," in manuscript in the Cambridge University Library. It appears to coincide very closely with other indications of his views, and it has been said of it, "There is much in it of the spirit both of Locke and Butler—of Locke in the spirit of observation and geniality; of Butler in the clear utterances as to the supremacy of reason, and the necessity of living according to our own true nature." The general principles of his regard of the Divine Being may be judged from the following extract : " Wherefore, to this eternal, infinitely good, wise, and powerful Being, as I am to pay all that adoration, thanks, and worship which I can raise up my mind unto; so to Him, from the consideration of His providence, whereby He doth govern the world, myself and all things in it, I am to pray for all that good which is necessary for my mind and body, and for diverting all those evils which are contrary to their nature; above all desiring that my mind may be endowed with all manner of virtue. But in requesting things relating to my body and its concerns, having always a deference to the will of the Supreme Being, who knows what is best for me better than I do my-

self. And though my requests to these bodily concerns
of mine are not answered, nevertheless, herein I worship
Him, by declaring my dependence upon Him; and for-
asmuch as that, in many respects, I have transgressed
His divine laws written upon my nature, I am humbly
to implore His pardon, it being as natural for me to do
it, as it is to implore the pardon of a man whom I
know I have offended. In all which requests of mine,
and all His creatures, how many soever they be in
number, and how distant soever they be in place, He
being infinite, is as ready at hand to hear and to help
as any man who is but finite is at hand to administer
food to his child that craves it."

Thus we take leave of Sydenham, denominated by
Locke "one of the master-builders at this time in the
commonwealth of learning;" reckoned by the masters
in his own and the next age as second to Hippocrates
alone—the man whom Boerhaave never mentioned to
his class without lifting his hat, describing him as
" Angliæ lumen, artis Phœbum, veram Hippocratici
viri speciem."

CHAPTER IV.

THE MONROS, CULLEN, THE GREGORYS, JOHN BELL, AND THE FOUNDATION OF THE EDINBURGH SCHOOL OF MEDICINE.

NOTWITHSTANDING the early date of the foundation of the College of Physicians of London, and the
fact that the illustrious names of Harvey and Sydenham
and others adorn the rise of rational medicine in the
south, the credit of first developing a famous medical
school belongs to Edinburgh, where the Monros, Gregorys,
Cullen, Black, and Rutherford maintained during the
eighteenth century an unbroken succession of brilliant
names. It cannot be allowed, however, that the Town
Council of Edinburgh, in founding medical professorships, deserves as much of this credit as do the outside founders of medical teaching, whose existence and
success extorted from the municipality a recognition
formal and limited at first, and certainly unremunerated.
It may be questioned whether the University of Edinburgh has not really been indebted almost as much to
the extra-academical teachers of medicine who have
continually stimulated the actual professors to their
best endeavours, as to those professors themselves.

Anatomy, the necessary foundation of medicine, had a kind of beginning in Edinburgh in 1505, for the surgeons and barbers of the city had procured the insertion in their charter of a clause enabling them to obtain "once in the year a condemned man after he be dead to make anatomy of." But little came of this, and it was reserved for a number of able physicians, educated abroad, in the latter part of the seventeenth century, to set on foot some practical teaching in medicine and the allied sciences. The names of Sir Robert Sibbald, Sir Andrew Balfour, and Sir Archibald Stevenson must be honourably mentioned in this connection. The first two of these were most influential in establishing the earliest public botanic garden in Edinburgh, a piece of ground about forty feet square, belonging to Holyrood House. They subsequently allied to themselves James Sutherland, who afterwards became a notable botanist, and obtained the appointment of keeper of a much larger garden near Trinity College Church. Many valuable collections of seeds and plants were procured; medical students were incited to collect and send home seeds and cuttings from places they might travel to ; and so the garden became an important starting-point for materia medica.

Professional feuds already became prominent in Edinburgh. The surgeon-apothecaries were jealous of the physicians and doctors of medicine. Several abortive efforts were made by the latter towards the establishment of a College of Physicians. In 1621 King James

gave a warrant to the Scottish Parliament for this purpose; but no action was taken. In 1630 the subject
was referred to the Privy Council. In 1656 Cromwell
constituted a College of Physicians for Scotland; but
his death prevented its completion. Thus it was not
till Sibbald and Stevenson, by the aid of Sir Charles
Scarborough, Harvey's friend, gained the ear of the
Duke of York, that at last the College of Physicians of
Edinburgh was founded, in 1681, notwithstanding the
strong opposition of the surgeons and the townsmen.

Soon after this, in 1685, the Town Council of
Edinburgh appointed three principal members of the
College of Physicians to be Professors of Medicine in
what they now for the first time, at any rate in existing
documents, called "the university of this city." Sir
Robert Sibbald was appointed Professor of Physic, and
rooms were allotted to him, but not a salary. Drs.
Halket and Pitcairne were speedily added to the list
of professors, and the division of duties between the
professors was left to themselves. We have no record
of any lectures given by these professors for a long
period, but we know that Pitcairne in 1692–3 held a
professorship at Leyden. On his return to Edinburgh
he became enthusiastic in promoting the medical
school, aiding Alexander Monteith in gaining permission from the Town Council to dissect the bodies of
people who died in "Paul's Work." "We offer," says
Pitcairne, "to wait on these poor for nothing, and bury
them after dissection at our own charges, which now

the town does; yet there is great opposition by the chief surgeons, who neither eat hay nor suffer the oxen to eat it. I do propose, if this be granted, to make better improvements in anatomy than have been in Leyden these thirty years."

Monteith obtained a grant in October 1694 of "those bodies that die in the correction-house," and of "foundlings that die upon the breast." He was allowed to make his dissections in "any vacant waste-room in the correction-house, or any other thereabouts belonging to the town." Magistrates were to be admitted if they desired, and the apprentices of the surgeons might attend at half-fee. However, Monteith's scheme did not succeed, because he had acted without concert with the other members of the Surgeons' Corporation. These made a more successful start in the same year, having obtained a right to "the bodies of foundlings who die betwixt the time that they are weaned and their being put to schools or trades, also the dead bodies of such as are stifled in the birth, which are exposed and have none to own them; also the dead bodies of such as are *felo de se* and have none to own them; likewayes the bodies of such as are put to death by sentence of the magistrate and have none to own them." A condition was annexed to this grant that by Michaelmas 1697 an anatomical theatre should be built, where public dissections should be made once a year, if opportunity offered. This was evidently intended to extend to a course of anatomy, including as much as could be taught on one body. The method, however, in which anatomy was first practised in the Surgeons' Hall was for ten surgeons to lecture, on following days, each in succession taking a special part. The body had to be buried within ten days.

It was in 1705 that a special appointment of one man to lecture on anatomy was first made, and the first lecturer, Robert Elliot, was also made Professor of Anatomy in the University, with a small stipend. This formal appointment appears to have been directly occasioned by the offer of some unknown teacher to give public and private teaching in anatomy to the surgeons and their apprentices.

It is not till 1706 that we have any record of Sibbald's lectures. The *Edinburgh Courant* was then made the medium whereby he announced, in Latin, his intention to lecture on natural history and medicine "in privatis collegiis," or private courses of lectures. He appears to have lectured in Latin, and to have received no pupils but such as were skilled in Greek, Latin, mathematics, and philosophy.

About this time had settled in Edinburgh the progenitor of the long line of distinguished Monros, John Monro, formerly an army surgeon, who became President of the College of Surgeons in 1712. His son Alexander, afterwards so distinguished, was born in London on the 8th September, 1697. Being an only son, his father gave unusual attention to his training, and early perceiving his acuteness of mind, sent him successively to London, Paris, and Leyden to obtain the best medical education at that time accessible. The anatomical preparations which he made during his studentship gave such evidence of ability, that Drummond, who then taught anatomy at Edinburgh, offered to resign in his favour as soon as he returned home. Cheselden in London and Boerhaave in Leyden were highly impressed by the young Scotchman's promise.

The year 1720 may be taken as witnessing the actual start of the Medical School of Edinburgh, and Alexander Monro as its real founder. Although the father did much to promote the successful start, the son becoming actually the competent teacher, must necessarily have the greater credit. At the age of twenty-two, Monro was appointed Professor of Anatomy, and having announced his first course of lectures on anatomy, to be illustrated by the preparations he had made and sent home when abroad, his father, without his knowledge, invited the President and Fellows of the College of Physicians and the whole of the city surgeons to the first lecture. The surprise caused the young lecturer to forget the discourse which he had committed to memory, and being without notes, he had presence of mind enough to commence talking about some of his preparations, and soon became collected in speaking of what he was confident he understood. Thus the surprise and temporary forgetfulness thereby caused was a foundation of his success : he found himself applauded as a ready speaker, and resolved throughout life to speak extempore, being persuaded that words expressive of his meaning would always occur in speaking on a subject which he understood. From this time the subjects of anatomy and surgery in Monro's hands attracted large classes of students, the average of the first decade being 67; of the second, 109; of the third, 147. Even during the second session his lectures attracted students from all parts of Scotland, also from England and Ireland. Seizing the opportunity, other professors were persuaded to start courses of lectures, so that soon a respectable curriculum was provided, and Monro secured in 1722 a grant of his professorship for life. It had previously been held only at the will of the Town Council.

Monro was now face to face with the difficulty of providing sufficient material for the instruction of his large classes. Under Cheselden in London he had been accustomed to a supply of subjects, more even than he could make use of. In Edinburgh, as early as 1711, complaints were made at Surgeons' Hall of violation of graves in Greyfriars' Churchyard, "by some who most unchristianly have been stealing, or at least attempting to carry away, the bodies of the dead out of their graves." But, said the surgeons, "that which affects them most, is a scandalous report, most maliciously spread about the town, that some of their number are accessory, which they cannot allow themselves to think, considering that the magistrates of Edinburgh have been always ready and willing to allow them what dead bodies fell under their gift, and thereby plentifully supplied their theatre for many years past." They consequently beg that the magistrates will seek for and punish the offenders, and resolve to expel any of their number found accessory to the violation of graves. The populace nevertheless continued to be excitable on the subject of the violation of graves, and in 1721–2, surgeons' apprentices were especially bound "not to raise the dead." In March 1725 Monro was put under the stringent obligation of giving information when he procured each dead body, and guaranteeing that it was regularly obtained; but the mob were suspicious, and threatened to demolish his museum and theatre at Surgeons' Hall. Monro consequently applied for and obtained a room in the university building, being there safer than at Surgeons' Hall. Here his course included dissections not only of the human body, but also of animals. Diseases affecting the various organs were referred to; operations upon the dead body were performed; bandages were applied; and lastly, such physiology as was known was treated of. This course was continued for nearly forty years.

A great hospital was lacking, and the whole force of the medical faculty, with the powerful aid of the far-seeing provost, George Drummond, was engaged to secure the building of the infirmary. Monro and Drummond were constituted a Building Committee, and Monro planned in particular the operation-room. Dr. Moore in his Travels through Scotland records that "the proprietors of many stone-quarries made presents of stone, others of lime; merchants contributed timber;

carpenters and masons were not wanting in their contributions; the neighbouring farmers agreed to carry
the materials gratis; the journeymen masons contributed their labours for a certain quantity of hewn
stones; and as this undertaking is for the relief of the
diseased, lame, and maimed poor, even the day-labourers
could not be exempted, but agreed to work a day in the
month gratis toward the erection. The ladies contributed
in their way to it; for they appointed an assembly for
the benefit of the work, which was well attended, and
every one contributed bountifully."

The completion of the hospital gave Monro the
opportunity of delivering clinical lectures on surgery,
while Rutherford from 1748 gave clinical lectures on
medical cases. Monro himself was present at every
post mortem examination, and dictated to the students
an accurate report of the case. It was said of him "it
is hardly possible to conceive a physician more attentive to practice, or a preceptor more anxious to communicate instruction."

His first and perhaps best known work was his
Osteology, published in 1726, and translated into
several foreign languages. A French edition appeared
in folio with excellent engravings by M. Sue, demonstrator to the Royal Academy of Paris. A treatise on
the Nerves followed; and later, a series of Medical
Essays and Observations, many by Monro, was issued
by him, as the result of meetings of the principal
medical men in Edinburgh, which flourished for some

years. Another interesting work of Monro's was his treatise on Comparative Anatomy, in which he proposed to illustrate the human economy by the anatomy of such vertebrate animals as he knew. But the contrast is astonishing between Monro's knowledge and that of the present day. He divides quadrupeds into carnivorous and herbivorous; fowls into those that feed on grain and those that feed on flesh; fishes into those that have lungs and those that have not. He remarks that the fishes that have lungs differ very inconsiderably from an ox or any other quadruped, and are not easily procured; consequently he omits all account of them. Moreover, he says, "as the structure of insects and worms is so very minute, and lends us but little assistance for the ends proposed, we purposely omit them." He has a strangely unpenetrating view of the relation between an oyster and a sensitive plant. "What difference is there betwixt an oyster, one of the most inorganised of the animal tribe, and the sensitive plant, the most exalted of the vegetable kingdom? They both remain fixed to one spot, where they receive their nourishment, having no proper motion of their own, save the shrinking from the approach of external injuries." Dr. Monro's writings generally are not inviting to quote from, being written in a plain and rather bald style, with very little attempt at illustration.

In private life Monro, primus, was humane, liberal in sentiment, a sincere friend, and an agreeable companion, an affectionate husband and a kind father, having the art of making his children his companions and friends. In 1745, after Prestonpans, he went down at once to the battlefield to assist the sick and wounded, dressed their wounds, and busied himself in securing them provisions and conveyance to town. Nor did he confine his attentions to the loyal, but aided the rebels also. He took an important share in the education of his children, of whom Donald became a successful physician, and wrote his life prefixed to the quarto edition of his works, 1781, to which all subsequent biographies are much indebted.

Monro was a man of a strong muscular make, of middle height. Yet his constitution was considerably weakened in early life owing to his being too frequently bled. He was liable to attacks of chest affections throughout life, but died finally of a painful ulcer of the rectum and bladder, on July 10th, 1767. He had resigned his chair of anatomy to his son Alexander in 1759, but continued to practise and to attend the infirmary till the last. He bore his painful illness with fortitude and Christian resignation, and talked of his approaching death with the same calmness as if he were going to sleep.

"He was," says Professor Struthers, "an able and active, and at the same time a calm and placid man. He had family and friends influential and plenty, but the work he had to do was of a kind at which friends could only stand and look on. He had to do a new thing in

Edinburgh; to teach anatomy and to provide for the study of it, in a town of then only thirty thousand inhabitants, and in a half-civilised and politically-disturbed country; he had to gather in students, to persuade others to join with him in teaching, and to get an infirmary built. All this he did, and at the same time established his fame not only as a teacher but as a man of science, and gave a name to the Edinburgh School which benefited still more the generation which followed him."

Although we must depart from strict chronological order to do so, it will be more convenient to give here an account of the second Monro, who was born May 20th, 1733, and was early attracted to the study of anatomy, showing great perseverance and possessing a good memory. He soon became a very useful assistant to his father in the dissecting-room, and when the students grew too numerous for one lecture, his father deputed his son, at the early age of twenty, to repeat his course in an evening lecture to those who had failed to obtain admission in the morning. His father, seeing how successful his son was, petitioned the Town Council to have him appointed as his colleague and eventual successor, promising, if this were granted, to send his son to the best medical schools in Europe, and in every way to fit him for the post. This plan being carried out, young Monro took his M.D. degree at Edinburgh in 1755, and set out for a round of medical schools, London, Leyden, Paris, and

Berlin; in London he attended William Hunter; in Berlin he had the still greater advantage of living in the house of, and sharing the intimate instruction of, the great anatomist, Meckel—a truly good start for a promising career. On his son's return to Edinburgh in 1758, his father resigned his chair to him, and the son commenced by teaching quite novel views on the blood, controverting his father's teaching. "The novelty of his matter, combined with the clearness of his style, is described by one who was present as having acted like an electric shock on the audience. It was at once seen that he was master of the subject, and of the art of communicating knowledge to others; his style was lively, argumentative, and modern, compared with that of his more venerable colleagues; and from the beginning onwards, for half a century, his career was one of easy and triumphant success" (Struthers). As a lecturer he was clear, earnest, and impressive, eloquent without display, and at the same time grave and dignified. No wonder that his classes increased in size, until they even reached four hundred.

At the same time Monro entered into practice as a physician, and became one of the leading practitioners in Edinburgh, so much so that Dr. James Gregory described him as being far more than half a century at the head of the medical school, and for a great part of that time at the head of the profession as a practising physician. He was also frequently called into consultation on surgical cases, though he did not operate. His chief fame is, however, as a successful anatomist and teacher of anatomy. In 1777 he successfully resisted the appointment of a separate Professor of Surgery, claiming that his office included surgery.

Monro secundus claimed, and not without good grounds, to have made important original discoveries in regard to the lymphatic system; but his merits as a discoverer in this department do not interfere with the greater lustre of William Hunter and Hewson. His observations on the structure and functions of the nervous system enjoy the distinction of having called Sir Charles Bell's attention to the ganglion of the fifth pair of cranial nerves, and to important particulars of the origin of the spinal nerves, which led in no insignificant degree to his own great discoveries.

In 1758 Monro published at Berlin his first essay on the Lymphatics, and Professor Black testified to having read this essay in manuscript in 1755. It contained an account of the lymphatics as a distinct system of vessels, having no immediate connection with the arteries and veins, but arising in small branches from all cavities and cells of the body into which fluids are thrown, and stating that their use was to absorb the whole or the thinner parts of these fluids, and to restore them to the general circulation. He showed further by medical observation that in cases where acrid matter was applied to the pores of the skin, or gained access to the cellular membranes, the glands between the parts affected and the centre of the body became swollen and painful, manifestly from being absorbed by the lymphatics.

Monro also first ascribed the absorption of bones and other solid parts in cases of tumour to pressure. His various works on the Nervous System, on the Muscles, on the Brain, Eye, and Ear, and on the Structure and Physiology of Fishes, all contain observations which were of considerable value in building up the science of anatomy in the last century, but none of them furnish attractive reading, such as we have found in the works of Harvey and Sydenham. This is somewhat remarkable, considering that Monro shone as an anecdotist, was intimate with all the celebrated Edinburgh men of his time, and was a great admirer of the theatre, being equally attracted by Mrs. Siddons, whom he felt the greatest pleasure in attending as a patient, and by Foote, whose performance as President of the College of Physicians to Weston's Dr. Last under examination he enjoyed extremely. It was said that Monro sent his own scarlet robe to the theatre for the mock doctor to wear.

Another of Monro's personal tastes was that of horticulture. He planted and beautified several romantic hills around his estate at Craiglockhart. Here he fitted up, says Dr. Duncan, a rural cottage, consisting of two commodious apartments, adjoining his head gardener's house, whose kitchen could provide dinner for a few select friends. He would keep no bedroom there, that he might never be tempted to stay away from his professional duties in Edinburgh; but in his cottage he often passed a summer day and regaled his friends with the choicest fruits. Dr. Duncan in his Harveian Oration relates his disappointment that the younger generation of his friends "prefer the instrumental music of a fiddle, a flute, or an organ in a drawing-room to that of the linnet, the thrush, or the goldfinch in the fields;" and that the gardens of his old friends in which he had spent such happy hours were now let out for market gardens.

Monro was very economical of his time, and carefully measured it out to each subject which occupied him; and he worked nearly as hard towards the end as at the beginning of his career. He did not deliver stereotyped lectures, but continually improved them. He is to be credited also with having favourably received Jenner's discovery of vaccination, and vaccinated many children himself.

In person the second Monro was of middle height, of vigorous and athletic make. His head was large, with strongly marked features and full forehead, light blue eyes, and somewhat large mouth. His neck was short, and his shoulders high.

In 1798 his son, Monro, tertius, was conjoined with him in the professorship, but for ten years more the old man continued to give the greater part of the course. His last lecture was that introductory to the session of 1808–9, after which he retired from practice also, and lived on till he died of apoplexy, 2d October 1817, in his eighty-fifth year.

Born to a great name and a ready-made position, as Professor Struthers remarks, the second Monro had every advantage which education, friends, and place could secure. But it is to his credit that among brilliant colleagues like Cullen, Black, Dugald Stewart, Playfair, and others, he held his own both intellectually and socially, even if he has not left so abiding a mark upon medical and anatomical science as his contemporaries must have expected him to make.

Notwithstanding the note which the Monros have attained for their anatomical teaching, and the distinction won by the Gregorys as Professors of Medicine and able physicians, they are outshone by William Cullen, who is justly the most conspicuous figure in the history of the Edinburgh Medical School in the eighteenth century. WILLIAM CULLEN was born on the 15th of April, 1710, at Hamilton, Lanarkshire, his father having been factor to the Duke of Hamilton. Early prominent at the local grammar-school by his quick perception and retentive memory, he was sent to the University of Glasgow in due course, and apprenticed to a medical practitioner named Paisley, who was both studious and possessed a good medical library, a signal advantage to young Cullen. It became remarked by his companions that while he took little or no part in their discussions when he happened to be ill-informed on the subject, he always so studied it afterwards that he could surpass the best of them if it came up again. At the close of 1729 Cullen went to London, and first obtained the surgeoncy to a merchant ship, commanded by a relative, with whom he went to the West Indies, remaining six months at Porto-bello. On his return to London he took a situation in an apothecary's shop in Henrietta Street, and studied as diligently as ever, when not occupied in the shop. His father had died, and there was little provision for a large family; his eldest brother's death compelled him to return to Scotland in the winter of 1731–2, to make arrangements for the education of his younger brothers and sisters. He began practice at Auchinlee near Hamilton, taking charge of the health of a relative, and perseveringly carrying on from books those studies which he had not money to prosecute at the seats of learning where he longed to be.

The receipt of a small legacy was the turning-point of Cullen's earlier fortunes: and how small a sum a studious Scotchman can make available in this direction is well known. Cullen resolved to devote himself to study entirely until he should be qualified to take a firm stand as a surgeon at Hamilton. He first went to reside with a dissenting minister in Northumberland, for the study of literature and philosophy, and then spent the winter sessions of 1734–5 and 1735–6 at Edinburgh Medical School, now rapidly rising into note. On establishing himself as a surgeon at Hamil-

ton early in 1736, young Cullen was soon employed
by the Duke and Duchess of Hamilton and the leading
families of the neighbourhood. In this comparatively
retired situation Cullen yet gained the confidence of
Dr. Clerk, an able Edinburgh physician called in to
Hamilton Palace, and was the means of influencing
William Hunter to the choice of the medical profession. William Hunter was Cullen's resident pupil
from 1737 to 1740, and declared these to have been
the happiest years of his life. Thus natural selection
brings men of future note together before the world has
known them, and the lineal succession of minds is as
fruitfully carried on as that of bodies. The affection
of these two continued throughout life. Long after
William Hunter refers to him as " a man to whom I
owe most, and love most of all men in the world."

Cullen determining to devote all his time to
medicine, proceeded to the M.D. degree at Glasgow in
1740, and took a partner who was to relieve him of
surgical work. In November 1741 he married Miss
Anna Johnstone, a lady of much conversational power
and charming manners, whose companionship he enjoyed for the long period of forty-six years. She became the mother of seven sons and four daughters. Dr.
Cullen's name was now becoming known considerably
beyond his native locality, and in 1744 he removed to
Glasgow, a step which he would have taken previously
but for the solicitations and promises of the Duke and
Duchess of Hamilton. His constant attendance on the

duke in his painful illness was ended by the death of the latter in 1743, which put an end to the project of a chemical laboratory and a botanical garden at the palace, which had been among the inducements by which he had been prevailed upon not to quit Hamilton. Henceforth, in the intervals of practice and study, he began to occupy himself vigorously with the founding of a medical school at Glasgow. He at once began to lecture on medicine, and subsequently added to his courses chemistry, materia medica, and botany, in all of which he gave lectures not merely representing the knowledge of the time, but also including original views of high value. The young school grew, though not so rapidly as that of Edinburgh; but thus early he was brought into contact with yet another great man, Joseph Black, who was for some years his intimate pupil, and afterwards left Glasgow for Edinburgh. Cullen discerned the promise of his pupil, and carefully abstained from entering upon fields of research in which he expected him to make a mark. Black submitted his treatise on fixed air to Cullen, and dedicated it to him. About this time Cullen made some important discoveries on the evolution of heat in chemical combination, and the cooling of solutions, some of which were not published till 1755, while others remained in manuscript, but suggested to Black important points in his view of latent heat.

At the beginning of 1751, by the interest of the Duke of Argyll, Dr. Cullen succeeded Dr. Johnstone as Professor of Medicine in the University of Glasgow, at the same time that Adam Smith was appointed to the Chair of Logic; and a friendship of great intimacy arose between these thoughtful minds. Only a few months afterwards, Adam Smith's transfer to the Moral Philosophy chair led Dr. Cullen to favour strongly the election of David Hume to the vacant chair, on an occasion when Edmund Burke was also a candidate. Neither was elected, strict orthodoxy carrying the day. At this period the applications of chemistry to arts and manufactures and to agriculture engaged Cullen's attention considerably, and he proposed to carry out a process for purifying common salt, but it proved too expensive.

Cullen, finding that Glasgow did not promise to build up a large medical school at present, and being compelled to take country practice, began to look longingly to Edinburgh, to which also his friends were calling him. He says in a letter to William Hunter, in August 1751, "I am quite tired of my present life; I have a good deal of country practice, which takes up a great deal of time, and hardly even allows me an hour's leisure. I get but little money for my labour; and indeed by country practice, with our payments, a man cannot make money." Various circumstances, however, prevented this step being taken, until, in the beginning of 1756, he was appointed to the professorship of chemistry at Edinburgh, and was thus fairly launched on his notable career. In the competition for this chair, Joseph Black had been nominated, but the two friends honourably refused to do anything to prejudice each other, and on appointment indeed Cullen offered Black all the fees if he would assist him. Cullen's first course at Edinburgh was attended by only 17 students, his second by 59, while it rose later to 145. Practice soon came to him, and freed him from his pecuniary struggles.

In 1757 Dr. Cullen first undertook to give clinical lectures in the infirmary, and in this work his especial talents shone. He had now had sufficient experience of practice, with the best knowledge of chemistry and materia medica that the time afforded; and his skill in observation and graphic description of disease, added to his zeal for imparting knowledge, soon made his clinical lectures renowned. In these lectures, for eighteen years most carefully prepared, the first real model of what is now so familiar to medical students as a clinical lecture was afforded. His candour may be judged from the following expressions: " In these lectures, however, I hazard my credit for your instruction, my first views, my conjectures, my projects, my trials, in short, my thoughts, which I may correct and if necessary change; and whenever you yourselves shall be above mistakes, or can find anybody else who is, I shall allow you to rate me as a very inferior person. In the meantime I think I am no more liable to mistakes than my neighbours, and therefore I shall go on in telling you of them when they occur." Pro-

moted by such candour, Cullen's reputation rapidly
grew. His lectures were remarkable for simplicity,
ingenuity, and comprehensiveness of view, with
copiousness of illustration. He taught his students to
observe the course of nature in diseases, to distinguish
between essential and accidental symptoms, and to
carefully discriminate the influence of remedies from
the curative operations of nature. "There is nothing,"
he said, "I desire so much as that every disease we
treat here should be a matter of experience to you, so
you must not be surprised that I use only one remedy
when I might employ two or three; for in using a
multiplicity of remedies, when a cure does succeed, it
is not easy to perceive which is most effectual." Again,
he says, "Every wise physician is a dogmatist, but a
dogmatical physician is one of the most absurd animals
that lives. We say he is a dogmatist in physic who
employs his reason, and, from some acquaintance with
the nature of the human body, thinks he can throw
some light upon diseases and ascertain the proper
methods of cure; and I have known none who were
not dogmatists except those who seemed to be incapable of reasoning, or who were too lazy for it. On the
other hand, I call him a dogmatical physician who is
very ready to assume opinions, to be prejudiced in
favour of them, and to retain and assert very tena-
ciously, and with too much confidence, the opinions or
prejudices which he has already taken up in common
life, or in the study of the sciences." He sought to

build up rational views of medicine, indeed, on the basis of fact and experiment. In giving his clinical lectures he was at great pains to choose diseases of the most common types, as most useful to the students. He adhered to great simplicity of prescriptions, compared with the complex and barbarous nostrums of preceding times, and he experimentally used and introduced many new drugs of great value, such as Cream of Tartar, Henbane, James's Powder, and Tartar Emetic.

The novelty with which Cullen invested his subject and the boldness of his views made many, especially conventional practitioners and lecturers, regard him with disfavour, and decry him for not regarding Boerhaave's views as final, and for adopting those of Hoffmann in conjunction with his own. Yet his lively and entertaining lectures, combined with his pleasing treatment of patients, and "his manner, so open, so kind, and so little regulated by pecuniary considerations, made him win his way more and more. He was the friend of every family he visited." William Hunter writes in 1758, "I do assure you I have never found anything in business so pleasing to me as to hear my patients telling me, with approbation, what Dr. Cullen had done for them, and to hear my pupils speaking with the reverence and esteem of Dr. Cullen that is so natural to young minds."

As a sign of the general mental attitude of Dr. Cullen, the following extract from a letter to his son James, on setting out for a foreign voyage, is of interest :

"Study your trade eagerly, decline no labour, recommend yourself by briskness and diligence, bear hardships with patience and resolution, be obliging to everybody, whether above or below you, and hold up your head both in a literal and figurative sense." While he aided his juniors in the best sense to acquire independence of character, he "admitted them freely to his house; conversed with them on the most familiar terms; solved their doubts and difficulties; gave them the use of his library; and, in every respect, treated them with the affection of a friend and the regard of a parent. It is impossible for those who personally knew him in this relation," says Dr. Aikin, "ever to forget the ardour of attachment which he inspired." Another and not less pleasing view of Cullen is shown in his recommendation of "Don Quixote" to Dugald Stewart when a boy suffering from some indisposition, and the interest he manifested in his patient's progress in that delight. He used to talk over with the lad every successive incident, scene, and character, manifesting the minutest accuracy of recollection of the master-piece.

We shall not follow the discussions which arose at Edinburgh about the succession to Dr. Rutherford's chair of the Practice of Physic, nor the circumstances which led to Dr. John Gregory's appointment. Suffice it to say that on the death of Dr. Whytt, Cullen consented to accept the chair of the Theory of Physic in 1766, and that subsequently an arrangement was made by which the two professors lectured alternately on the Theory and Practice of Physic, to the still greater advantage of the now celebrated school. This appointment was strongly promoted by both the Monros, and by an address signed by 160 medical students. The arrangement now made lasted till Dr. Gregory's death in 1773, when Cullen became sole Professor of the Practice of Physic. Black was brought to Edinburgh to succeed Cullen in the Chair of Chemistry.

Cullen's principal works are the "Nosology," a synopsis and classification of diseases, with definitions, which obtained wide popularity, although only an approximation to a sound system; and his "First Lines of the Practice of Physic," 4 vols., 1778–85, which went through numerous editions. One of its especial merits was that it pointed out more clearly than preceding works the extensive and powerful influence of the nervous system on disease. It is now held as the defect of his system that it was too theoretical, and that its views were not adequately supported by facts. It cannot be denied that Cullen had but moderate anatomical and physiological knowledge, and this has prevented him from leaving works capable of being read with much profit by the practitioners of the present day.

It is after all on William Cullen's personal influence on the School of Medicine, which he did so much to maintain, that his fame will chiefly rest. The character of this influence is honourable and stainless. Dr. James Anderson has left in unequivocal language a record of his bearing in his conspicuous position which does equal honour to his intellectual energy and to his qualities of heart. Dr. Cullen, he says, was employed five or six hours a day in visiting patients and prescribing by letter; lecturing never less than two hours a day, sometimes four; yet, when encountered, he never seemed in a hurry or discomposed—always easy, cheerful, and sociably inclined. He would play at whist before supper with as keen interest as if a thousand pounds depended on it.

Cullen did not leave his acquaintance with his students to originate by chance, but invited them early in their attendance, by twos, threes, and fours, to supper, and gaining their confidence about their studies, amusements, difficulties, hopes, and prospects. Thus he got to know all his class, and paid especial attention to those who were most assiduous, best disposed, or most friendless. He made a point of finding out who among them were most hampered by poverty, and often found some polite excuse for refusing to take a fee even for their first course, and in many cases for their second course. One method he adopted was to express his wish to have their opinion on a particular part of his course which had been omitted for want of time the previous session, and he would thereupon present them with a ticket for the second course. After two courses he did not require any fee for further attendance. He is credited, too, with having introduced into Edinburgh the practice of not taking fees for medical attendance on students of the university. This ease and generosity about money matters was the cause of his eventually dying without any fortune. It is said that he used to put sums of money into an open drawer, to which he and his wife went when they wanted any.

We shall not enter here into the controversy between Dr. John Brown, founder of the Brunonian theory of medicine, and his disciples, and Dr. Cullen, to whom Brown had owed everything in his youth. Brown's system proved to be no more stable than his personal character, although its noisy advocacy, and the abuse heaped upon him personally, caused Dr. Cullen much pain.

Cullen continued to deliver his lectures until 1789, having resigned his professorship on the 30th December, and he died on the 5th February 1790, almost eighty years of age. He was buried at Kirknewton, in which parish was situated his estate of Ormiston Hill. This latter, which he had beautified with very great care, had to be sold after his death for the benefit of his family.

Dr. Anderson describes Dr. Cullen as having a striking and not unpleasing aspect, although by no means elegant. His eye was remarkably vivacious and expressive. In person he was tall and thin, stooping very much in later life. In walking he had a contemplative look, scarcely regarding the objects around him. When in Edinburgh he rose before seven, and would often dictate to an amanuensis till nine. At ten he commenced his visits to patients, proceeding in a sedan chair through the narrow closes and wynds. He always lived, while in Edinburgh, in a comparatively small house in the Mint, not far from the seat of his academical duties. For them he may be said to have lived and died.

The family of the Gregorys has been perhaps equally celebrated with the Monros in connection with university life in Scotland, and has certainly furnished it with a larger number of eminent professors. James Gregory, the celebrated inventor of the reflecting telescope, was the first great man of the family, and his publication of a work on optics in 1663 marked an era in that science. His early death in 1675, at the age of 37, deprived science of many brilliant discoveries in prospect. His only son, James, became Professor of Medicine in King's College, Aberdeen, and died in 1731.

His younger son, JOHN GREGORY, the first of the medical Gregorys who became associated with the fame of Edinburgh, was only seven years old when his father died in 1731. After being educated at Aberdeen, under the care of his elder brother, who had succeeded his father, and also under the influence of his cousin, Thomas Reid, the well-known metaphysician, young Gregory entered at Edinburgh in 1741, and studied under the elder Monro, Sinclair, and Rutherford; and at the Medical Society commenced a warm friendship with Mark Akenside, author of the "Pleasures of Imagination." In 1745–6 he studied at Leyden under

Albinus, and having received the M.D. degree from Aberdeen during his absence, he was elected to the chair of philosophy there on his return, and lectured there for three years on mathematics, and moral and natural philosophy. In 1749 he resigned this chair in order to devote himself to medicine, and in 1752 he married Elizabeth, daughter of Lord Forbes, who had beauty, intellect, and wit, and brought him a fortune.

Finding that Aberdeen afforded him no sufficient field for practice in competition with his elder brother, Gregory went in 1754 to London, where he had already friends such as Wilkes and Charles Townshend, whom he had met at Leyden, and where he speedily made other friends, of whom may be mentioned George, Lord Lyttelton, Edward and Lady Mary Wortley Montagu. He was at once elected into the Royal Society, and would no doubt have gained fashionable support; but his elder brother dying in 1755, he was recalled to Aberdeen to fill the Professorship of Medicine. Here he continued to practise and to lecture till 1764, publishing in the latter year "A Comparative View of the State and Faculties of Man with those of the Animal World." He then removed to Edinburgh with a view to securing a professorship there. This fell to his lot in 1766, on the death of Rutherford. In the same year he succeeded Dr. Andrew Whytt as physician to the king in Scotland. He at first lectured on the Practice of Physic solely, but in 1770 he agreed with Cullen that they should lecture in alternate years on the

Theory and the Practice, and this arrangement was continued permanently. As a lecturer he was very successful, simple and not in any way oratorical in style. He was especially noted for some lectures on the "Duties and Qualifications of a Physician," which were afterwards published, and went through several editions. He gave the profits to a poor and deserving student. In 1772 he published "Elements of the Practice of Physic," a kind of syllabus of lectures; and this completes the list of his medical works. His name was more known after his death as the author of a little book of advice to young girls, "A Father's Legacy to his Daughters," which has gone through very many editions. His tone may be judged from the following extract:—

"Do not marry a fool; he is the most untractable of all animals; he is led by his passions and caprices, and is incapable of hearing the voice of reason. . . . But the worst circumstance that attends a fool is his constant jealousy of his wife being thought to govern him. This renders it impossible to lead him; and he is continually doing absurd and disagreeable things, for no other reason but to show he dares do them. . . . A rake is always a suspicious husband, because he has known only the most worthless of your sex. He likewise entails the worst diseases on his wife and children if he has the misfortune to have any."

Gregory's predominant qualities were good sense and benevolence. In conversation he had a warmth of

tone and of gesture that were very pleasing, united to
gentleness and simplicity of manner. To his pupils
he was a friend, ever easy of access, and ready to
assist them to the utmost. His Edinburgh life was
spent in intimate association with David Hume, Lord
Monboddo, Lord Kaimes, Dr. Blair, and the elder Tytler.
James Beattie loved him with enthusiastic affection, as
the closing stanzas of "The Minstrel" testify. Gregory
died suddenly on the 9th February 1773, from gout,
from which he had frequently suffered. He had thus
scarcely attained the age of fifty.

JAMES GREGORY, who succeeded his father in the professorship, was born in Aberdeen in 1753. He was
educated in Edinburgh, and also studied for a short
time at Christ Church, Oxford, where his relation, Dr.
David Gregory, had been dean. He acquired a strong
taste for classics and no little classical erudition, so
that he was throughout life fond of making apposite
Latin quotations, and wrote that language easily and
accurately. He was still a student of medicine at
Edinburgh when his father's sudden death took place
in 1773. The son by a great effort completed his
father's course of lectures, and showed so much ability
that the professorship was practically kept open for
him. In 1774 he took the M.D. degree, and spent the
next two years in studying medicine on the Continent.
In 1776, being then only twenty-three, he was
appointed Professor of the Institutes of Medicine, and
in the following year also commenced to give clinical

lectures at the infirmary, which method of instruction he continued for more than twenty years. His practice at first was not extensive, until his pupils had themselves become practitioners, and called him in as a consultant. In his later years, after Cullen's death, his practice increased largely, and in the ten years preceding his death he had the leading consulting practice in Scotland.

In 1780–2 Gregory published his "Conspectus Medicinæ Theoreticæ," written in excellent Latin; it speedily became widely known, and was extensively read not only in Britain but also on the Continent. It has gone through numerous editions. Its more important and valuable portions were those dealing with therapeutics. In 1790 he was appointed Cullen's successor in the chair of the Practice of Medicine, and from that time continued to lecture to large classes down to his death in 1821 (April 2). Thus he held an almost autocratic position for the long period of over thirty years; and it is much to be regretted that his great talents in repartee, quick memory for telling quotations, and fondness for a joke, led him to take an active part in the medical controversies which have embittered so many careers in Edinburgh. The long list of controversial books and pamphlets by Dr. Gregory, given by Mr. John Bell in his "Letters on Professional Controversy and Manners," 1810, could be considerably extended, and it affords a melancholy picture of misplaced energy. One of these extended to 700 pages quarto, and its tone may be judged from the following extracts from the "Memorial to the Managers of the Royal Infirmary."

"Let us suppose that in consequence of this memorial, every individual member of the College of Surgeons shall, to his own share, make forty times more noise than Orlando Furioso did at full moon when he was maddest, and shall continue in that unparalleled state of uproar for twenty years without ceasing. I can see no great harm in all that noise; and no harm at all to any but those who make it. . . . Ninety-nine parts in the hundred of all that noise would of course be bestowed on me; whom it would not deprive of one hour of my natural sleep, and to whom it would afford infinite amusement and gratification while I am awake."

"We are certainly a most amiable brotherhood, as every person must acknowledge who has had the good luck to see but a dozen and a half or two dozen of us together, especially if he saw us at dinner. Yet, whatever the majority of us may be, I am afraid we are not all perfect angels. Some of us at least appear to be made of the same flesh and blood, and to be subject to the same frailties and passions and vices as other men. The consequence is, that when two or three of us are set down together in a little town, or fifty or a hundred of us in a great town, and obliged to scramble for fame, and fortune, and daily bread, we are apt to get into rivalships, and disputes, and altercations which sometimes end in open quarrels and implacable animosities, to the very great annoyance of those who are, and the no less entertainment of those who are not, our patients. A consultation among any number of such angry physicians or surgeons in all probability will conduce as little to the benefit of their patient as a congress of an equal number of game-cocks turned loose in a cock-pit, for probably the good of the patient will be the last and least object of their thoughts."

Inasmuch as he takes occasion to say of John Bell, "any man, if himself or his family were sick, should as soon think of calling in a mad dog as Mr. John Bell," we can judge of the position in which any one found himself who had the misfortune to displease Dr. Gregory. We must believe, however, on the testimony of many who knew him, that he must have possessed many remarkable and excellent qualities to have won so large a share of their attachment and esteem as he undoubtedly did. Dr. Alison says of him (Encyc. Brit., 8th ed.), that the boldness, originality, and strength of his intellect, and the energy and decision of his character, were strongly marked in his conversation, and that he showed both warm attachment to his friends, and a generosity almost bordering on profusion. He disdained to conciliate public favour, and often gave unrestrained vent to a strongly irascible temper. He would not give up his point in argument, and would overwhelm his opponents with quotations, jests, and satire.

As a teacher Gregory was conspicuous for a sound practicality. He highly approved of a maxim which he often brought forward: "The best physician is he who can distinguish what he can do from what he cannot do." Pathology in his days was a very rudimentary science, and hence he distrusted all theories in regard to the essential nature of disease as premature and visionary. He was at home in the study of diagnostic and prognostic symptoms, and paid considerable attention to the action of remedies. He had no tendency to meddlesome medicine, restraining and discountenancing treatment when there was no hope or prospect of success. He believed strongly in the antiphlogistic or lowering treatment of inflammatory diseases, and in the use of preventive measures in warding off the attacks of chronic diseases. Thus he presented the spectacle of an advocate of temperance, of bodily exertion without fatigue, and of mental occupation without anxiety, who by no means followed his own prescriptions.

As a lecturer he displayed a most ready command of language, and an excellent memory especially for cases he had seen, the details of which he could accurately remember from the name alone of the patient. He gained great influence over the minds of his pupils, not merely by the humour and the abundance of his illustrations, but also by the outspoken exposition of his views and his commanding energy. His frankness showed itself too in the candour with which he communicated his opinions to the relatives or friends of his patients. He took a genuine interest in his patients, and convinced them of his sincerity, notwithstanding a certain roughness of manner. Where he felt no personal antagonism he was on very cordial terms with his professional friends, and succeeded in gaining their esteem and regard by his manner towards them in consultation. He was, as we have said before, the admitted autocrat of the profession in Edinburgh in his later years, and it is much to be regretted that his contributions to the science of medicine are so few.

Gregory used to say that while physic had been the business, metaphysics had been the amusement of his life. Reid dedicated jointly to him and to Dugald Stewart his " Essays on the Intellectual Powers ; " and he was an attached friend of Thomas Brown, and interested himself greatly in securing his succession to Dugald Stewart in the chair of Moral Philosophy. He went so far in philology as to publish a Theory of the Moods of Verbs in the "Edinburgh Philosophical Transactions" for 1787. His "Literary and Philosophical Essays," in two volumes, (1792), dealt mainly with the old controversy as to Liberty and Necessity. However, since he had a strong opinion that metaphysics admits of no discoveries, it is not surprising that his contribution to the science failed to secure a permanent place. His fourth son, William Gregory, became a distinguished chemist, the friend of Liebig and translator of his

"Familiar Letters on Chemistry," and Professor of Chemistry in the University of Edinburgh.

JOHN BELL, who comes last to be mentioned in the list of great Edinburgh men of the eighteenth century, is linked with the nineteenth in part by his surgical career and posthumous "Observations on Italy," and still more by his relationship to his great brother, Sir Charles Bell. Every one who reads the scattered memorials of John Bell will be filled with regret that his career should have been blighted by controversy and what appears even malignant opposition, led by Dr. James Gregory. His artistic tastes and acquirements, combined with his original views on anatomy and surgery, made him a specimen of a new genus in Edinburgh, and it is certain that Edinburgh did not adequately appreciate him.

John Bell, the second son of the Rev. William Bell, a clergyman of the Scottish Episcopal Church in Edinburgh, was educated for the medical profession by his father's choice, in gratitude for the relief he had received by means of a difficult surgical operation about a month before his son's birth, in 1763. He was apprenticed to Alexander Wood, a well-known surgeon in 1779, for five years. He attended the lectures of Black, Cullen, and the second Monro, and became a fellow of the Edinburgh College of Surgeons in 1786. Monro not being an operating surgeon, John Bell saw many defects in his teaching as to the applications of anatomy to surgery. In fact, surgical anatomy was never adequately taught in Edinburgh till he himself commenced to teach, and actual dissection was little thought of. He says, "In Dr. Monro's class, unless there be a fortunate succession of bloody murders, not three subjects are dissected in the year. On the remains of a subject fished up from the bottom of a tub of spirits are demonstrated those delicate nerves which are to be avoided or divided in our operations; and these are demonstrated once at the distance of one hundred feet, nerves and arteries which the surgeon has to dissect, at the peril of his patient's life." *

Immediately after qualifying, therefore, John Bell commenced lecturing on anatomy and surgery on his own account, an audacious proceeding which did not fail to draw down upon him the antagonism of all those who stood by the old lines. He was vigorous in his denunciation of the stereotyped methods and imperfections of the old school of Monro and Benjamin Bell. He built a house for his courses and practical work in Surgeons' Square, where he carried on his work after 1790. He soon came into popularity, and this increased as his style became more polished and formed, being in fact the most graphic which had appeared in the Edinburgh Medical School. He was a masterly descriptive writer, and used all the charms of style to give interest to his subject. Consequently his opponents said that he romanced and exaggerated.

* "Letters on the Education of a Surgeon," by John Bell, 1810.

He stuck to his text that surgery must be based upon anatomy and pathology; and unfortunately aroused the bitterest opposition of James Gregory, who first published an anonymous pamphlet entitled "A Guide to the Medical Students attending the University of Edinburgh," warning students against attending John Bell's lectures. The next attack was a "Review of the Writings of John Bell, Surgeon in Edinburgh, by Jonathan Dawplucker." This malignant attack, says Bell, was stuck up like a playbill, in a most conspicuous and unusual manner, on every corner of the city; on the door of my lecture-room, on the gates of the college, where my pupils could not but pass, and on the gates of the infirmary, where I went to perform my operations.

Bell replied by adopting the nickname used by his opponent, at the same time attacking his surgical ally in conventional methods, Benjamin Bell, whose "System of Surgery," in six volumes, afforded him excellent sport. Bell says, "I neither mistook my bird, nor missed my shot; and on the day in which the second number was published, the great surgical work of Benjamin fell down dead." At this time it was customary for all the surgeons of Edinburgh who cared to do so to operate in rotation at the infirmary, and Gregory put forward a plan by which only a select and limited number of surgeons were to be allowed this privilege. But the scheme was especially aimed at securing the exclusion of John Bell, and this Gregory accomplished in 1800. However, Bell had gained notoriety and practice, though he had lost the hospital appointment, and apparently all chance of a university professorship. He gave up teaching, and devoted himself to practice. He had been instrumental in raising the tone of university requirements and theories in his branch, and it could not again sink to its former inferior condition. He became the leading operator and consulting surgeon of his time. "He was not only a bold and dexterous operator," says Professor Struthers, " but combined all the qualities, natural and acquired, of a great surgeon, to an extraordinary degree. He was original and fearless, and a thorough anatomist; he had intellect, nerve, and also language— was master alike of head, hand, and tongue or pen; and he was laborious as well as brilliant." Generous himself and liberal to those who were necessitous, he knew how to reprove niggardliness in the wealthy. On one occasion a rich Lanarkshire laird gave him a cheque for £50 for services which Bell considered to deserve much higher remuneration. On reaching the outer door he met with the butler, and said to him, " You have had considerable trouble opening the door to me, there is a trifle for you," and gave him his master's cheque. The astonished butler of course consulted his master about this mark of doubtful favour, and the laird, understanding the hint, sent after the skilful surgeon a cheque for £150.

John Bell has, however, other claims to remembrance than his teaching and his operative skill. His anatomical and surgical writings are still worthy of consultation, and aided materially in the progress of the science. His principal works of this class were the "Anatomy of the Human Body," 3 vols. (1793–1802); "Engravings of the Bones, Muscles, and Joints," illustrating vol. i. of the Anatomy, 1794; "On the Nature and Cure of Wounds," 1795; and "Principles of Surgery," 3 vols., 1801–8. Sir Charles Bell speaks of "the rapid improvement in the surgery of the arteries which followed the publication of this part of the Anatomy:" and further, that it could not easily be surpassed for correctness and minuteness of description. The third volume of the Anatomy was by his brother Charles, under whose subsequent editorship the book went through numerous editions, and was translated into German. The treatise on Wounds contained clear expositions of the novel practice of aiming at the early union of wounds after operations, and also emphasised the importance of the free anastomosis of arteries in all cases where injuries were sustained by the main arterial trunks. In his "Principles of Surgery" he gave excellent historical views of his subject, as well as the latest and best practice founded on anatomy and physiology. Sir Charles Bell makes the following pointed contrast between his brother and Sir Astley Cooper, in regard to their methods: "He (John Bell) seems ever most happy when he can support his reasoning by the authority of those who have preceded him, and feels that he has conferred a double benefit when he can at the same time illustrate the truth and vindicate the character of some excellent old surgeon, and teach the youth of the present day to look back to the history of the profession for their most useful lessons. Sir Astley Cooper, on the other hand, hates all authority which interferes with his popularity; votes that volume to be an old musty one which is dedicated to himself; omits all mention of his respectable contemporaries; and only varies his terms of praise and eulogy on the young men whom he flatters, journalists and connections in business, down to the cutler who makes his instruments."

In 1805 John Bell married Rosina Congleton, daughter of a retired Edinburgh physician, and in her found congeniality of tastes, an appreciation of the artistic, literary, and musical sides of his nature, and admirable assistance in his propensity for exercising hospitality. His entertainments, and his own performances on the trombone, became celebrated. His taste for art was accompanied by remarkable skill in design and execution, in which he was only excelled among surgeons by his own brother Charles. He never, however, felt quite at ease after his exclusion from the infirmary. His rivals occupying their position of authority, Dr. Gregory in perpetual sway, could not but impress him with a sense of undeserved failure. Early in 1816 he was thrown from his horse, and did not recover rapidly from his injuries. In 1817 his health was so much impaired that he went on a foreign tour with his wife, and his last three years were spent in Italy, where his artist soul found great delight, and where he also had much professional practice among English visitors to Italy.

During his residence in Italy he was well aware of the dangerous condition of his health, but his singular degree of spirit and ardour of character prevented his ever betraying his consciousness of it. A few pencilled lines, written by him before leaving Paris, express well the inmost heart of the man whose career had presented such outward turbulence. He says: "I have seen much of the disappointments of life. I shall not feel them long. Sickness, in an awful and sudden form; loss of blood, in which I lay sinking for many hours, with the feeling of death long protracted, when I felt how painful it was not to come quite to life, yet not to die—a clamorous dream! tell that in no long time that must happen, which was lately so near." He died of dropsy, at Rome, on April 15, 1820.

In Florence and Rome he visited all the principal galleries, and took pencil notes of his observations, both from a scientific and artistic point of view. These formed the main bulk of his posthumous "Observations on Italy," edited by his friend, Bishop Sandford of Edinburgh, published in quarto form in 1825, subsequently in 2 vols. 8vo in 1835, with additional chapters on Naples. On their publication they at once took high rank, from their singular combination of artistic sympathies, literary expression, and scientific criticism. The *New Monthly Review*, on its first page, described the language of these observations as vigorous, terse and pure; his lights and shadows as disposed with a masterly hand. His descriptions both of landscapes and of manners in Italy are referred to as the most fascinating that had yet appeared. As a specimen of this vivid and picturesque style, showing how much his art was aided by that quickness to perceive characteristic expressions and traits which was so trained by his medical experience, we may quote his account of a Lenten preacher whom he heard at Rome.

" A sandal-footed, bare-armed, unclothed-looking monk, young, with a pale visage and negligent aspect, stood leaning against a pillar at the upper end of the middle nave; his grey coarse habit, girded by various folds of thickly-knotted cords, seemed scarcely to cover his person; his almost naked arms hanging down by his side, while his cowl, which had fallen back, discovered a wild pallid countenance, and a long lean bony throat. He stood silent and motionless, like an image or statue, as if lost in meditation, or exhausted by the vehemence of his own overwrought feelings poured out upon his auditors. The orator had evidently reached to an elevated strain before my entrance, leaving, as he had suddenly paused, vivid traces of the force of his arguments on the countenances of those he addressed. Here the spread hands, the half-opened mouth, the strained eye, spoke an earnest yet amazed attention, while perhaps near him stood, with silvered hair and meek aspect, the pale anchorite, trembling while he listened, lest perchance even he might not be secure against the punishments of the evil-doer: while beyond him might be seen the dark, gloomy, steady gaze of the brooding fanatic, whose flashing eye seemed to kindle with the orator, and keep pace with his denunciations,—perhaps contrasted by the quiet unthinking air of contented stupidity, looking as if the sense of hearing alone were roused, or by the speaking eye, beaming with zealous fire, as if ready to challenge or answer each new proposition. Some stood with downcast looks, serious and reflecting; others walked softly along, now seen, now lost among the pillars; while the larger portion, who had been as it were surprised by their emotion into a momentary taciturnity, were hastily forming into groups, and beginning, in whispered accents, to converse with that eagerness and vivacity which so peculiarly characterise their nation. But soon, above those murmuring sounds, the full deep-toned voice of the preacher struck the ear, when suddenly all was again hushed to silence. Slow and solemn he opened his discourse; but, as he proceeded, his features became gradually more animated; his dark deep eloquent eye kindling as he spoke, and throwing momentary radiance over his wan and haggard countenance, while the round mellow tones of the Italian language gave the finest energy to his expressions. With frequent pauses, but with increasing power, he continued his discourse; his voice now low and solemn, now grand and forcible, but still with moderated and ever-varied accents, which worked on the feelings, at one moment producing the chill of strong emotion, and then, as he changed his tone, melting the heart to tenderness. The object of his sermon and self-imposed mission was to gain votaries, and win them to a monastic life, by portraying the dangers, the turbulence, and the sorrows of the worldly, contrasted with the peaceful serenity of the heaven-devoted mind. Occasionally, as if warmed by a pro-phetic spirit, with an air now imploring and plaintive, now wild and triumphant, with animated gesture and tossing of the arms, alternately pointing to heaven and to the shades below, he seemed as if he would seduce, persuade, or tear his victim from the world. The powers of his voice and action gave an indescribable force to his language, carrying away the minds of his auditors with a rapidity that left no pause for reflec-tion. The sombre chastened light of day bringing forward some objects in strong relief, and leaving others in shade, the peculiar aspect of the monk, the magic influence which seemed to hang on his words and lend force to his eloquence, gave to the whole scene a character at once singular and striking."

John Bell was below middle stature, of good figure, active, with regular features, keen penetrating eyes, and highly intellectual expression. His widow says of him: "To a classical taste and knowledge of drawing (many of his professional designs being finely executed by his own hand) he joined a mind strongly alive to the beauties of nature. He would often, in his earlier years, yield to the enjoyment they produced, and, wandering among the wild and grand scenery of his native land, indulge his imagination in gazing on the rapid stream or watch the coming storm. Such habits seem to have tended, in some measure, to form his character; training him especially to independence in judgment, and perseverance in investigation, that led him to seek knowledge, and boldly publish his opinions. With warm affections and sanguine temper, he looked forward with the hope that his labours and reputation would one day assuredly bring independence; and meanwhile, listening only to the dictates of an enthusiastic nature, and yielding to the impulse of feeling, he would readily give his last guinea, his time, and his care, to any who required them. Judging of others by himself, he was too confiding in friendship, and too careless in matters of business; consequently from the one he was exposed to disappointment, and from the other involved in difficulties and embarrassments which tinged the colour of his whole life."

CHAPTER V.

*WILLIAM AND JOHN HUNTER AND THE APPLI-
CATIONS OF ANATOMY AND PHYSIOLOGY TO
SURGERY.*

IT is somewhat surprising that anatomy, the necessary
basis of a sound treatment of the human body in
disease, should have so long remained comparatively
uncultivated in this country as a practical art, after
Harvey had led the way and shown how brilliant
discoveries might be made by dissection. Continental
schools certainly put to shame early English efforts in
anatomy : and it would appear not easy to establish in
England any new study, unless the subject is one from
which large pecuniary profits may immediately be
anticipated—in which enterprise there can be no sort
of merit. When a man has attained some reputation
as an anatomist or physiologist, all the efforts of British
society seem to be directed towards taking him away
from that pursuit of which he has proved himself an
ornament, and converting him into a man whose
business it is to cure private ailments, thereby preventing him but too successfully, in most instances, from

pursuing that for which he has shown conspicuous talent. Thus we find Cheselden, whose publication of an Anatomy of the Human Body, in 1713, and Osteography in 1733, had shown great anatomical ability, was carried into a large private practice. And William Hunter, the founder of the first great anatomical museum, was diverted from his proper studies to become an obstetrician, in order to obtain money for his special objects.

WILLIAM HUNTER, whose name has been previously mentioned in our account of Cullen, was born on May 23, 1718, at Kilbride, Lanarkshire, being the seventh of ten children of John and Agnes Hunter. At fourteen he was sent to Glasgow for his education, remaining there five years, it being his father's wish that he should enter the Church. Imbibing liberal opinions, he soon became averse to this proposal, and his intimacy with Dr. Cullen determined his thoughts towards medicine. In 1737 he became Cullen's resident pupil at Hamilton, and remained with him three years. It was then agreed that he should go and study medicine at Edinburgh and London, and afterwards return to Hamilton to a partnership with his master. Their mutual attachment was lifelong.

The winter of 1740–1 was spent by William Hunter at Edinburgh, where Monro primus was then teaching anatomy. The following summer he went to London, and obtained the position of assistant to Dr. Douglas, who was then engaged on a great book on osteology,

which he did not live to complete, the education of Dr.
Douglas's son being also placed in his charge. He
considered this offer so inviting that he remained in
London, although it was contrary to the wishes of his
now aged father, who thought the arrangement with
Dr. Cullen preferable. The father died on the 30th
October following, aged 78.

The young man soon became expert in dissection,
and he entered as a surgeon's pupil at St. George's
Hospital. His prospects were soon after clouded by
the death of Dr. Douglas, but his residence in the
family was not interrupted. As early as 1743 he
communicated to the Royal Society a paper on the
Structure and Diseases of Articulating Cartilages; and
thereafter was occupied in preparing to commence teaching anatomy. His opportunity came in 1746, when
Mr. Samuel Sharpe gave up a course of lectures on
surgery, which he had been delivering to a society of
navy surgeons in Covent Garden, and recommended
William Hunter in his place. His lectures were found
so satisfactory that they asked him to extend his course
to anatomy. He had great timidity in lecturing at
first, but soon gained confidence. One of his pupils
who accompanied him home after his introductory
lecture, relates that he carried his fees for the course,
amounting to seventy guineas, in a bag under his cloak,
and that he remarked that it was a larger sum than he
had ever been master of before. The profits of these
courses he expended in no niggardly spirit, to a large

extent in befriending others, and he was consequently
unable to begin his next season's lectures at the proper
time, owing to lack of means to advertise their commencement.   He learnt a salutary lesson by this delay,
for he found that by so far straining his resources he had
only encouraged the idleness of his friends.   This made
him for the future cautious of lending money, and more
economical than before, and may be said to have laid
the foundation of his fortune.

In 1747 William Hunter was admitted a member of
the College of Surgeons, and in the spring took a continental journey, in which he met Albinus at Leyden.
Although he commenced practice as a surgeon, he
gradually discontinued it when he began to succeed
as an accoucheur, being appointed surgeon-accoucheur
to both the Middlesex Hospital and the British Lying-
in Hospital.   His conciliating manners and pleasing
address contributed to make him popular in this
branch of practice.   In 1750 he obtained the degree of
M.D. from the University of Glasgow, and about the
same time ceased to reside with Mrs. Douglas, and
went to Jermyn Street, so long associated with the
Hunters.   In 1751 he visited his home at Long Calderwood, Kilbride, and gratified his affection for Dr.
Cullen, who had now become established at Glasgow.
As Cullen was one day riding with him, he pointed
out to Hunter how conspicuous Long Calderwood was
from a distance, when the latter replied with energy,
" Well, if I live, I shall make it still more conspicuous."

This, however, was his only visit to his native place after his settling in London.

William Hunter joined the College of Physicians in 1755, and the Medical Society about the same time. His "History of an Aneurism of the Aorta," appears in the first volume published by that Society, in 1757. In regard to aneurisms he had made many original observations, such as to place the subject in a totally new aspect. Several papers he contributed to this Society bear directly on problems of interest in midwifery and the diseases of women.

It was in 1762 that the first edition of the "Medical Commentaries" appeared, in which Monro secundus was severely attacked for having claimed as his own discoveries which William Hunter had, years before, promulgated at his lectures. It is to be regretted that in regard to these very matters, as well as others, disputes afterwards arose between William Hunter and his brother John, who it appears had made at least some of these discoveries, while engaged as assistant to his brother. In respect of a number of these, the elder brother gave credit to his junior both when lecturing and in his publications; in regard to others, the elder gave no credit at all when John conceived himself entitled to much, or all, of the praise of originality. Both brothers were strikingly sensitive as to their claims to originality, and William Hunter on several occasions seems to have regarded a new demonstration as his property because made in his dissecting-room, though not by himself. Yet we find it recorded that in the winter 1762–3, when the brothers had separated, William Hunter would frequently say in his lectures : "In this I am only my brother's interpreter "—"I am simply the demonstrator of this discovery ; it was my brother's." We must recur to this subject later, merely mentioning now, that John Hunter acted as his brother's assistant and dissected for him from 1748, and that from 1755 to 1760 a certain portion of the lectures was delivered by him ; in 1760 they separated.

There is no question that in general education, in manners, in delivery, in all that makes the successful lecturer and the attractive practitioner, William Hunter greatly excelled his brother. Dr. Baillie has said of him, " No one ever possessed more enthusiasm for his art, more persevering industry, more acuteness of investigation, more perspicuity of expression, or indeed, a greater share of natural eloquence. He excelled very much any lecturer whom I have ever heard in the clearness of his arrangements, the aptness of his illustrations, and the elegance of his diction." If it were not for the tenacity with which he pursued controversial topics, and his unfortunate disagreement with his brother, there would be nothing to mar the pleasurable nature of the picture of William Hunter. The way in which he himself viewed this side of his character may be gathered from the following extract from the Supplement to his Medical Commentaries, published in 1777.

" It is remarkable, that there is scarce a considerable character in anatomy, that is not connected with some warm controversy. Anatomists have ever been engaged in contention. And indeed, if a man has not such a degree of enthusiasm, and love of the art, as will make him impatient of unreasonable opposition, and of encroachments upon his discoveries and his reputation, he will hardly become considerable in anatomy, or in any other branch of natural knowledge.

" These reflections afford some comfort to me, who unfortunately have been already engaged in two public disputes. I have imitated some of the greatest characters, in what is commonly reckoned their worst part : but I have also endeavoured to be useful; to improve and diffuse the knowledge of anatomy : and surely it will be allowed here, that if I have not been serviceable to the public in this way, it has not been for want of diligence, or love of the service.

" It has likewise been observed of anatomists, that they are all liable to the error of being severe on each other in their disputes. Perhaps from being in the habit of examining objects with care and precision, they may be more disgusted with rash assertions, and false reasoning. From the habit of guarding against being deceived by appearances, and of finding out truth, they may be more than ordinarily provoked by any attempt to impose upon them ; and for anything that we know, the passive submission of dead bodies, their common objects, may render them less able to bear contradiction."

It would have been pleasing if we could have related that William Hunter allowed supreme merit to any one anatomist or physiologist who preceded him. But we find him saying about Harvey : " In merit, Harvey's rank must be comparatively low indeed. So much had been discovered by others, that little more was left for him to do, than to dress it up into a system ; and that, every judge on such matters will allow, required no extraordinary talents. Yet, easy as it was, it made him immortal. But none of his writings show him to have been a man of uncommon abilities." Dr. Hunter must surely have been aware that this was carping criticism, for on a preceding page he had spoken of Harvey as a first-rate genius for sagacity and application.

The years after his brother's secession brought Dr. Hunter to the summit of professional success. His obstetric knowledge and skill were known to be so great that he was called in to consultation respecting the Queen in 1762. Two years later he was appointed physician extraordinary to her majesty. His increasing engagements soon left him little time for his dissecting-room and lectures, and he engaged as assistant one of his pupils, William Hewson, and afterwards took him into partnership in his lectures. But this connection was severed, owing to disputes, in 1770, and Hewson commenced lecturing on his own account,

and achieved great success, which was cut short, however, by his early death from fever in 1774. Cruickshank was his successor with Dr. Hunter, and continued his partner till the death of the latter.

In 1768, the year after his election into the Royal
Society, William Hunter was appointed the first Professor of Anatomy to the newly-founded Royal Academy, and he entered upon this field of work with
great vigour, applying his anatomical knowledge to
painting and sculpture with his usual success. On
the death of Dr. Fothergill he was elected President
of the Society of Physicians, now the Medical Society
of London.

The most remarkable work which William Hunter
published was a great series of folio plates of the Human
Gravid Uterus, begun in 1751, and published in 1775.
In the dedication of this work to the King he acknowledged that in most of the dissections he had been
assisted by his brother, " whose accuracy in anatomical
researches is so well known," he says, " that to omit
this opportunity of thanking him for that assistance
would be in some measure to disregard the future
reputation of the work itself." But this acknowledgment did not content John Hunter, who claimed the
original merit of most of the discoveries his brother
announced, and communicated a full account to the
Royal Society in 1780, five years after his brother's
work was published. At the next meeting of the
Society William Hunter replied to his brother's claims,

and John rejoined. The consequence was that the Society published nothing on the subject, but retained the papers of both in manuscript. The anatomical description of William Hunter's plates was completed by his nephew, Dr. Baillie, and published in 1794.

A still more important work, as regarded costliness, was the formation of the museum, which still remains for the benefit of students as the Hunterian Museum in Glasgow University. Economical from the first, as regarded his personal expenses, William Hunter, after laying aside a sufficient sum to provide for old age or sickness, applied his thoughts to the foundation of an anatomical school in London. During Mr. Grenville's administration, in 1765, he petitioned him for the grant of a piece of ground on which to build an anatomical theatre, undertaking to spend £7000 on the building, and to endow a permanent professorship of anatomy. It can hardly be believed that such a munificent offer was rejected ; but it was the middle of the eighteenth century, and the government pension to Dr. Johnson was probably considered the utmost stretch of public countenance to learning and science. Lord Shelburne, it is true, expressed a wish that Dr. Hunter's proposal might be carried out by means of a general subscription, and offered himself to contribute a thousand guineas. But William Hunter was not the man to depend for the execution of his projects upon an appeal of this kind, and he consequently purchased a plot of ground in Great

Windmill Street, near the Haymarket, where he built a suitable house for his own residence, with a lecture-theatre, dissecting-rooms, and a handsome room for a museum. To this he removed in 1770 from Jermyn Street. He had already a very large collection of human, comparative, and morbid anatomy, which he continued to augment. He purchased all the best collections of morbid and other anatomical specimens that were offered for sale, such as those of Sandys, Falconer (which included Hewson's), and Blackall. To these were added numerous specimens of rare diseases, presented to him by medical friends and pupils. We discern the light in which he viewed these gifts by the following statement in one of his publications: " I look upon everything of this kind which is given to me as a present to the public, and consider myself as thereby called upon to serve the public with more diligence." And the museum was always open to the many visitors who were attracted by its fame.

Dr. Hunter's tastes expanded. He collected fossils, rare books, and coins. Dr. Harwood described his library as including the most magnificent treasure of Greek and Latin books that had been accumulated by any person then living. The anatomist even discovered a bibliographical novelty in comparing two copies of the Aldine edition of Theocritus, which he found to present material differences, though representing the same edition. The collection of coins in this museum was of such value and importance that an illustrated quarto was devoted to the description of a portion of them by William Combe. The preface gives an account of the progress of the collection, which had now cost no less than twenty thousand pounds.

Another important addition was made to the museum in 1781 in the shape of Dr. Fothergill's collection of shells, corals, and other natural history specimens. Dr. Fothergill's will directed that William Hunter should have the first refusal of the museum at five hundred pounds less than its value as ascertained by appraisement, and Dr. Hunter eventually made the purchase for twelve hundred pounds.

This noble museum was left by his will, not to his brother John, but to his nephew Dr. Baillie, and in case of his death to Mr. Cruickshank, for thirty years, at the end of which time the collection was to go to the University of Glasgow. Dr. Baillie, however, handed it over to Glasgow before the time specified. Eight thousand pounds was also left to keep up and increase the collection.

Dr. Hunter never retired from practice, although much tormented by gout in his later years. He thought at one time of settling down somewhere in Scotland, when suffering more than usual from ill-health, but having found the title of an estate offered him to be defective, and also having to provide for his constantly increasing museum expenses, he laid aside his intention. He continued most persevering both in his practice and in his lectures, notwithstanding his augmented sufferings, until on the 15th of March 1783 he was almost prostrated. On the 20th, however, he would deliver his lecture introductory to the operations of surgery, notwithstanding the dissuasions of his friends. Towards the end of his lecture he fainted, and had to be carried to bed by two servants. In the following night he had an attack of partial paralysis, from which he did not rally. During his illness he said to his friend, Mr. Combe, "If I had strength enough to hold a pen, I would write how easy and pleasant a thing it is to die." His brother John was admitted to see and attend him on his deathbed, and no hint of disagreement on these occasions is given. William Hunter died on the 30th March 1783, in his sixty-fifth year, and was buried at St. James's Church, Piccadilly.

William Hunter was of an elegant figure, slender, and rather below the middle height. The portrait of him by Sir Joshua Reynolds adorns the Hunterian Museum at Glasgow. An unfinished painting by Zoffany represents him in the attitude of lecturing on the muscles at the Royal Academy, surrounded by academicians. Hunter's portrait is the only completed part. It was presented to the College of Physicians by Mr. Bransby Cooper in 1829.

We hear of no matrimonial projects at any time on William Hunter's part. He was wedded to his museum, his profession, his lectures. He lived a

frugal life, eating little food, and that plainly prepared; rising early, and being always at work. When
he invited friends to dine with him, he seldom provided more than two courses, and he often said, " A
man who cannot dine on one dish deserves to have
no dinner." A single glass of wine was handed after
dinner to each guest. Some accused him of parsi-
mony. The truth is that he did not relish the
amusements and luxuries in which most people indulge, but he was by no means parsimonious as to the
pursuits in which he found real pleasure. His biographer, Dr. Foart Simmons, says: "There was something very engaging in his manner and address, and
he had such an appearance of attention to his patients
when he was making his inquiries as could hardly fail
to conciliate their confidence and esteem. In consultation with his medical brethren, he delivered his
opinions with diffidence and candour. In familiar
conversation he was cheerful and unassuming. All
who knew him allow that he possessed an excellent
understanding, great readiness of perception, a good
memory, and a sound judgment."

Dr. Hunter made no bequest to his brother John;
but he knew that the latter was well established and
successful. Still, his bequest of the family estate at
Long Calderwood to his nephew, Dr. Baillie, appears
not to have been altogether satisfactory to the latter,
who handed it over to his uncle John. Dr. Hunter
left an annuity of £100 to his sister, Mrs. Baillie, for

life, and £2000 to each of her daughters.   Dr. Baillie
was his residuary legatee.

The name of JOHN HUNTER recalls the glories of a
great medical school, the labours of an indefatigable
dissector, the skill of a brilliant operating surgeon,
and the formation of the noblest of the Hunterian
museums, that of Lincoln's-Inn-Fields, the richest
heritage of the London College of Surgeons.   The
youngest son of the same parents as William Hunter,
John was the child of his father's old age, the latter
approaching seventy at John's birth on February 13th,
1728.   The father died when John was ten years old,
and his mother appears to have been extremely indul-
gent to her youngest child, and so little controlled his
desires for amusements that he left the local grammar-
school almost destitute of classical knowledge, which
formed, of course, the staple instruction there imparted.
The imperfection of his general early education was a
painful drawback to John Hunter all his life.

There is no doubt that when about seventeen John
went to Glasgow on a visit to his sister, Mrs. Buchanan,
whose husband, a cabinet-maker, was failing to get on
in business, owing to his musical and social qualities.
How far John took part in the business is not recorded,
but it is likely that he owed much of his mechanical
skill to what he learnt at the shop, which seemed
to stick to him much more closely than any book-
learning.   Finding his efforts to relieve his sister

from her difficulties ineffectual, he returned home to
Long Calderwood. Mrs. Buchanan died in 1749.

We have extremely little knowledge of the workings
of John Hunter's mind in his youth, or how far he
was conscious of the great talents that were awaiting
the appropriate incentive. His being much given to
country amusements is all that we know. At length he
tired of having no profession, and his brother William's
success attracted him to London. He begged that he
might pay a visit to him, and be his assistant in anatomy, if possible. The request being acceded to, John
arrived in London in September 1748, was at once set
to work upon a dissection of the muscles of the arm to
illustrate his brother's lectures, and succeeded beyond
expectation. He was now established in his brother's
dissecting-room in the winter, and in the summer
attended Chelsea Hospital under Cheselden. It was
evident that John had found an occupation suited
to his capabilities, and in his second season he was
placed in full charge of the pupils in the dissecting-
room, while Dr. Hunter almost confined himself to
his lectures. In 1751 John became a pupil at St.
Bartholomew's Hospital, where Percival Pott was then
a leading surgeon. In 1754 he was entered as a
surgeon's pupil at St. George's Hospital, where a
chance of a surgeoncy was more likely than at St.
Bartholomew's. In 1756 he was for some months
house-surgeon at St. George's.

Between these two last dates he became temporarily

resident at Oxford, where his name was put down at
St. Mary's Hall, June 5, 1755. Probably the idea was
that he should become a physician, taking an Oxford
degree in medicine; but he was in no humour "to
stuff Latin and Greek at the University;" and he
never conquered his aversion to classics. Long afterwards he wrote: "Jesse Foot* accuses me of not
understanding the dead languages; but I could teach
him that on the dead body which he never knew in
any language dead or living." The last entry of
charges for battels against John's name in the buttery-
book of St. Mary's Hall occurs on July 25, 1755, so
that he probably resided less than two months. His
name was kept on the books, however, till December 10,
1756.

The only variation we hear of in his constant round
of work was a visit John paid to his home in 1752.
In 1755 John was admitted to a certain degree of
partnership in Dr. Hunter's lectures; besides undertaking a definite part of the course, he was to supply
his brother's place when absent on professional engagements. This was a serious source of discomfort; the
younger Hunter's defective education here became prominent. We may take a description of his style of
lecturing at a later period from his avowed enemy,
Foot, but it will be well to deduct one half from it as
the product of animosity. "In the beginning, these
lectures were written on detached pieces of paper; and

---

* Author of the defamatory so-called Life of John Hunter, 1794.

such was the natural confusion of his mind, that he would be frequently found incapable of explaining his own opinions, from his notes; and after having in vain tried to recall the transitory ideas, now no longer floating in the mind, nor obedient to the will—after having in vain rubbed up his face, and shut his eyes, to invite disobedient recollection—he would throw the subject by, and take up another."

Meanwhile, passing laborious days in the dissectingroom, John was becoming a more perfect anatomist than his brother, and began making discoveries on his own account, some of which William demurred to at first, but usually accepted and brought forward in his lectures, giving John credit for them. Among other discoveries of this time may be mentioned that of the ramifications of the nerves of smell in the nose, the unravelling of branches of the fifth nerve, previously unknown, the tracing of the arteries in the gravid uterus, and the existence of lymphatic vessels in birds. Other discoveries made by John Hunter are described in William Hunter's Medical Commentaries. But it soon appeared that the younger brother felt he did not receive a due share of praise and acknowledgment of his labours, while the elder considered every discovery made in his dissecting-room as more or less his property. John continued to dissect "with an ardour and perseverance of which there is hardly any example. His labours were so useful to his brother's collection, and so gratifying to his disposition, that although in many other respects they did not agree, this simple tie kept them together for many years " (Sir E. Home).

John gradually became led into the study of comparative anatomy, from finding that structures which were complex in the human subject were simpler in animals, or different in plan, in both cases throwing light on human anatomy and physiology. Thus he made dissections of all the commoner animals, and always preserved the parts which interested him. He soon passed beyond the ordinary range, and made acquaintance with the keeper of the Tower menagerie, that he might obtain the bodies of such animals as died there. Similarly he even would purchase animals when alive, from travelling showmen, simply requiring them to bring him their bodies whenever they happened to die. He bought all rare animals that came in his way : others were presented to him by friends, and thus an ample supply of material was secured.

There is some obscurity about the reasons which induced the younger brother in 1760 to accept an appointment as staff-surgeon in the army, joining the expedition to Belleisle in 1761. There is not much doubt, however, that his health had suffered, and that a foreign voyage and residence were calculated to restore him. In 1762 he was employed with the army in Portugal, and in this experience laid the foundation of his knowledge of military surgery. During this expedition he neglected no opportunity of forwarding his studies in comparative anatomy

and physiology. Thus when at Belleisle, in order to
discover whether animals in a state of hibernation could
digest food, he introduced worms and pieces of meat
into the stomachs of lizards, and kept them under
observation in a cool place. He found the substances
so introduced remained perfectly undigested. So in
1762, near Lisbon, he tested the hearing of fishes by
observing the effect of the report of a gun upon the
inhabitants of a nobleman's fish-pond.

Retiring from the army after the peace of 1763,
John Hunter found his place in his brother's dissecting-room occupied by Mr. Hewson, a most capable
dissector and lecturer. Hence he had no option but
to depend on his own exertions, and he started in
London practice as a surgeon in Golden Square. He
found that practice came but slowly, and formed a
class for the study of anatomy and practical surgery to
add to his income. This, too, never proved nearly so
remunerative as his brother's lectures, owing to John's
defects of style and expression already mentioned.
His success in practice was also retarded by his refusal
or failure to employ any of the arts or tact needed to
gain personal popularity. Although he was a good
convivial companion, at any rate in his earlier days,
any festive enjoyment was always subordinated to
his zeal for a new specimen or a rare case, from which
he could learn something. He would take any trouble,
or go any distance, with these ends in view; while his
feeling about an ordinary case may be gathered from a

remark to his attached friend, Lynn, as he laid aside his dissecting instruments—" Well, Lynn, I must go and earn this d—d guinea, or I shall be sure to want it to-morrow." Mere fashionableness Hunter could not tolerate. Dr. Garthshore, a physician of the old school, always formal, polite, and well dressed, accosting him one day in his dissecting-room with his usual *empressement*, " My d-e-a-r John Hunter,"—was astonished to hear the mocking reply, " My d-e-a-r Tom Fool." The busy dissector was not likely to value highly the formalities of the courtly doctor, who as a contemporary remarks, " occasionally looked in, wound up his watch, and fell asleep."

Finding his collection of live animals grow beyond his means of providing for them in town, Hunter purchased a considerable piece of ground at Earl's Court, then about two miles outside London, and built upon it a house with a lawn behind it, upon and around which he kept a collection of curious variety, and sometimes under comparatively slight control, in order that their habits might the more readily be watched. On one occasion two leopards got loose, and one was scaling the boundary wall, while the other was engaged in combat with dogs, when Mr. Hunter, unarmed, went out and seized them both and replaced them in their outhouse; an act of courage which, when it was over, nearly caused him to faint.

In 1767 an accident by which Mr. Hunter ruptured

his tendo Achillis, whether while dancing, or in getting up from the dissecting-table after being cramped by long sitting, is not certain, occasioned him to study carefully the process by which ruptured tendons are healed. His method of treating himself was to keep the heel raised, and to compress the muscle gently with a roller, thus preventing any spasmodic contraction. He divided the same tendon in several dogs, killing them subsequently at different periods to examine the progress and nature of the repair; and his experiments and specimens were the origin of the present practice of cutting through tendons for the relief of distorted and contracted joints.

In the same year, 1767, Mr. Hunter was elected into the Royal Society, before his brother—an evidence that his eager investigations were already making him well known to men of inquiring minds. At a later period he was one of the originators of meetings at a coffee-house to discuss papers before their submission to the Society generally. In 1768 he became a member of the Royal College of Surgeons, and in the same year, supported by his brother's interest, he was elected surgeon to St. George's Hospital by 114 to 42 votes. He was now in a position in which more patients were at his disposal for experimental or novel modes of treatment, and in which he could take resident pupils on advantageous terms. In 1770 his brother's removal to his new premises in Great Windmill Street, led to John's transfer to his brother's

late house in Jermyn Street, where he found much
more ample accommodation for his work than he had
hitherto possessed. Here among his earliest pupils
was Dr. Jenner, who was an enthusiastic disciple,
and whom Mr. Hunter would gladly have permanently associated with him. He kept up a continual
and intimate correspondence with him throughout life,
often asking Dr. Jenner for information on questions
of natural history.

Soon after his removal to Jermyn Street, namely,
in July 1771, Mr. Hunter married Anne, eldest
daughter of Mr. Robert Home, an army surgeon,
father of his subsequent pupil and associate, Sir
Everard Home. He had been engaged to Miss Home
for some years, but financial reasons had hitherto
postponed the marriage. Mrs. Hunter had artistic,
literary, and musical tastes, which to some extent, by
their expense, trenched on her husband's scientific
objects. She is remembered as the author of the
words of a number of Haydn's English canzonets,
including the celebrated one, " My mother bids me
bind my hair." Mr. Hunter sometimes found that
his wife's friends were too fashionable or frivolous
for his taste, and occasionally his irritation got the
better of his manners. It is related that once,
returning late in the evening after a wearisome day's
work, he unexpectedly found his drawing-room filled
with gay company, walked straight into the room, and
addressed the assembly in these terms: " I knew

nothing of this kick-up, and I ought to have been informed of it beforehand; but as I am now returned home to study, I hope the present company will now retire:" a hope speedily realised. Hunter much preferred the weekly social assemblies at which his scientific friends were welcomed, and where the conversation was pointed and informing. Still there is no ground for reflecting on the general happiness of Mr. Hunter's married life. Of his two children who survived infancy, he often said that if he had been allowed to bespeak a pair of children, they should have been those with which Providence had favoured him. His wife survived him till 1821, when she died in her 79th year.

Early in 1771 Mr. Hunter published his first work of any magnitude, the first part of his "Treatise on the Natural History of the Human Teeth," which long continued a standard work, largely appropriated by subsequent writers. The second part, treating of the diseases of the teeth, did not appear till 1778. In 1772 he made his mark at the Royal Society by his celebrated paper on the digestion of the stomach after death, which he attributed to the action of the gastric juice upon the dead tissues. His stores of knowledge and learning were afterwards made evident by many papers in the "Philosophical Transactions," of which the principal were those on the torpedo (1773), on the air receptacles of birds, and on the Gillaroo trout, 1774; the production of heat by animals and vegetables, 1775 ; the recovery of persons apparently drowned, 1776; the communication of smallpox to the fœtus in utero, 1780; the organ of hearing in fishes, 1782; the specific identity of the wolf, jackal, and dog, and on the structure and economy of whales, 1787 ; observations on bees, 1793; and on some remarkable caves in Bayreuth, and fossil bones found therein, 1794. The titles of these papers, however, convey but a very imperfect idea of the wide range of subjects treated in them. When he described a structure, he made it the starting-point of a dissertation, in the course of which he brought to bear all his vast stores of knowledge to establish general principles or to illustrate important points of physiology.

In the autumn of 1772 his brother-in-law, Everard Home, became his pupil. He describes Hunter's museum at this time as already having an imposing magnitude. All the best rooms in the house were devoted to it, and it was continually being enlarged by his unremitting toil. From six, or earlier, till nine, when he breakfasted, Hunter dissected; after breakfast till twelve he was at home to patients. Punctuality he observed to a fault. He would leave patients at home in order to start punctually to his outside consultations, " for," said he, " these people can take their chance another day, and I have no right to waste the valuable time of other practitioners by keeping them waiting for me." He kept one book at home in which to enter these, and had an exact

copy of it always in his waistcoat pocket: thus those
at home by referring to the book could invariably
find him. Once his former pupil, Cline, having to
meet Hunter in consultation, made a second arrangement, unknown to Hunter, to take him to see another
patient of his immediately after. Hunter's outburst
of passion at this unjustifiable disturbance of his
arrangements for the afternoon was with difficulty
appeased. His punctuality at dinner, at four, was
equally settled, but he strictly ordered that dinner
should be served whether he were at home or not.
For many years he drank no wine, and sat but a
short time at table, except when he had company;
but he nevertheless pressed the guests to disregard
his example. "Come, fellow," said he, in his usual
blunt way, to Mr., afterwards Sir William, Blizard,
"why don't you drink your wine?" The guest
pleaded in excuse a whitlow, which caused him
much pain. Hunter would not allow the validity of
the plea, but continued to urge him and ridicule his
excuse. "Come, come, John," said Mrs. Hunter,
"you will please to remember that you were delirious
for two days when you had a boil on your finger
some time ago." This turned the laugh against
Hunter, who ceased to importune his guest.

In addition to his own pre-eminent industry, Hunter
was not without the most important talent of making
others' labours advance his ends. Thus for fourteen
years he employed a very capable ycung artist named

Bell, keeping him resident in his house, occupied in making drawings, and anatomical preparations, and generally in museum work. Bell was frequently called in also to act as Hunter's amanuensis. After he left Mr. Hunter, in 1789, he became an assistant-surgeon under the East India Company, settling at Bencoolen, where his zoological studies were continued with much promise of great achievement; but, unfortunately for science, he died of fever in 1792.

In 1772 Hunter began to lecture on the theory and practice of surgery, at first to his pupils and a few friends admitted gratuitously, but afterwards on payment of a fee of four guineas. This may be accounted the first introduction into this country, perhaps to any, of the idea of principles of surgery, and the necessity of a rational explanation of processes of repair, and of a scientific basis for operations. Instead of a study of anatomy alone being required by a surgeon, he elevated pathology into its true position, and brought in all the aids with which physiology and comparative anatomy could at that time illuminate the subject. But in advance of any of these aids was his own clear insight, which penetrated to the core of a question, and often brought out truth which he could not himself explain, or only imperfectly. He never overcame his difficulty in lecturing; at the commencement of each course he always composed himself by a draught of laudanum. His lectures, delivered on alternate evenings from

October to April, were given from seven to eight o'clock. His class was usually comparatively small, never exceeding thirty; but the quality of his audience was good, as may be gathered from its having included Astley Cooper, Cline, Abernethy, Carlisle, Chevalier, and Macartney. He never became an attractive lecturer; from deficiency in extempore speaking, he was compelled to read his lectures, and seldom raised his eyes from his manuscript. His manner was frequently ungraceful, but his matter was for the most part highly intelligible and luminous to those of his hearers who came prepared by thought and attainments to be really edified, while he was often unintelligible to those who had no practice in thinking for themselves and desired to keep clear of that odious pain. In his lectures he was equally unsparing towards his own and others' errors, and he never clung to his own past opinions. "Never ask me," he replied to a question, "what I have said or what I have written ; but if you will ask me what my present opinions are, I will tell you."

The following extract from Ottley* gives an interesting view of Hunter's after-dinner habits. "After dinner he was accustomed to sleep for about an hour, and his evenings were spent either in preparing or delivering lectures, in dictating to an amanuensis the records of particular cases, of which he kept a regular

* "Life of John Hunter," by Drewry Ottley, 1835.

entry, or in a similar manner committing to paper
the substance of any work on which he chanced to
be engaged. When employed in the latter way,
Mr. Bell and he used to retire to the study, the
former carrying with him from the museum such
preparations as related to the subject on which
Hunter was engaged: these were placed on the table
before him, and at the other end sat Mr. Bell, writing
from Hunter's dictation. The manuscript was then
looked over, and the grammatical blunders, for Bell
was an uneducated man, corrected by Hunter. At
twelve the family went to bed, and the butler, before
retiring to rest, used to bring in a fresh Argand lamp,
by the light of which Hunter continued his labours
until one or two in the morning, or even later in
winter. Thus he left only about four hours for sleep,
which, with the hour after dinner, was all the time
that he devoted to the refreshment of his body.
He had no home amusements for the relaxation of
his mind, and the only indulgence of this kind he
enjoyed consisted in an evening's ramble amongst
the various denizens of earth and air which he had
congregated at Earl's Court."

In January 1776 Mr. Hunter attained a court
position, being appointed surgeon-extraordinary to
the king. In the same year he became interested in
the efforts of the Humane Society, and at its request
drew up a paper for the Royal Society on the
recovery of the apparently-drowned. Herein he

makes a just distinction between absolute death and
suspended animation, illustrates different modes of
dying, and describes many signs of life and death.
This year was also the first in which he delivered
the Croonian lecture to the Royal Society, on muscular
motion, a subject which he continued in successive
years till 1782 (omitting 1777); but the lectures were
never published, being, he said, too incomplete.

In the year 1773 Mr. Hunter suffered the first
open onset of the disease which occasioned him such
acute pain and distress for many years, in an attack
of spasm accompanied by cessation of the heart's
action apparently for three quarters of an hour.
During the attack, however, sensation and voluntary
actions were kept up, and he was able to continue
respiring by voluntary effort. In the next few
years the attacks were somewhat rare; but from 1783
onwards he was subject to severe angina pectoris
whenever mentally agitated. In 1777 a constant
giddiness or vertigo seized him on account of his
being called upon to pay a large sum of money for a
friend for whom he had become security, at a time
when it was exceedingly inconvenient to do so. This
illness led him to visit Bath in the autumn, leaving
Mr. Bell and Mr. Home to catalogue his museum.
At Bath Dr. Jenner visited him and was surprised at
his altered appearance, and here first diagnosed his case
as dependent upon an organic affection of the heart:
but he did not tell Hunter his diagnosis, fearing an

injurious effect. Returning to town, and soon recovering his usual health and vigour, Mr. Hunter published
in 1778 the second part of his Treatise on the Teeth,
dealing with their diseases. In 1779 a paper contributed to the Royal Society on the hermaphrodite
black cattle or free martin gave him occasion to describe hermaphroditism in general. In 1780 occurred
the unfortunate controversy with his brother, in regard
to the discovery of the utero-placental circulation, to
which we have already referred. The estrangement
which followed was extreme, and protracted till the
elder brother lay on his deathbed. After his brother's
death, however, which occurred just at the conclusion
of John Hunter's course of lectures, when he had
finished his lecture, he still seemed to have more to
say; and at length, appearing as if he had just recollected something, he began, "Ho! gentlemen, one
thing more: I need not remind you of ——: you all
know the loss anatomy has lately sustained." He was
obliged to pause and turn his face from his hearers.
At length recovering himself, he stated that Mr.
Cruickshank would occupy the place of Dr. Hunter.
This, and a few words more, were not spoken without
great emotion, nor with dry eyes. The scene was so
pathetic, that a general sympathy pervaded the class;
and though all had been preparing to leave, they
stood or sat motionless for several minutes.

The eagerness with which Mr. Hunter sought and
appropriated all rarities is amusingly illustrated by

his own remarks to Dr. Clarke, who had a preparation illustrating extra-uterine pregnancy, which Mr. Hunter often viewed with longing eyes. "Come, Doctor," said he, "I positively must have that preparation." "No, John Hunter," was the reply, "you positively shall not." "You will not give it me, then?" "No." "Will you sell it?" "No." "Well, then, take care I don't meet you with it in some dark lane at night, for if I do, I'll murder you to get it." It is reported that a specimen which remains one of the most valued in the Hunterian Museum cost Mr. Hunter no less than £500 in 1783, namely, the skeleton of O'Brien, the Irish giant, seven feet seven inches high. It appears that O'Brien had heard of and dreaded the scalpel of the famous dissector, and took special precautions to frustrate his ends. He made an Irish league with several compatriots that his body should be taken to sea, and securely sunk in deep water; but Mr. Hunter, more subtle than the giant, had made a big bargain with the undertaker, who arranged that during the funeral progress towards the sea the coffin should be locked up in a barn while its guardians were drinking at a tavern. The corpse was speedily extracted, and a sufficient weight of stones substituted; and Hunter soon rejoiced in the possession of his prize, which he drove to Earl's Court in his own carriage, and quickly converted into a skeleton.

In 1781 Mr. Hunter was called by the defence as a witness in the trial of Captain Donellan at Warwick

Assizes for the murder of his brother-in-law, Sir
Theodosius Boughton. In his evidence Mr. Hunter
gave all that could justly be deduced from the facts
known to him, but refused to speak positively as to
the cause of death. Under cross-examination he
became confused and hesitating, as was certain to be
the case. This rather aroused the wrath of Mr.
Justice Buller, who in his charge said, " I can hardly
say what his opinion is, for he does not seem to have
formed any opinion at all of the matter." But
Hunter's caution was undoubtedly justifiable.

In 1783 the lease of the Jermyn Street house
expired, and finding it difficult to accommodate his
museum in any premises he could obtain, Mr. Hunter
purchased the remainder of the lease, extending to
twenty-four years only, of a house on the east side of
Leicester Square, with ground extending on the rear to
Castle Street, where there was a second smaller house.
On the vacant ground Mr. Hunter determined to build
a museum for his collection, including a large upper
room fifty-two feet by twenty-eight, lighted from
above, and having a gallery running round it. A
lecture-room and other rooms were beneath. By the
spring of 1785 this considerable undertaking was complete, absorbing all Hunter's spare cash and costing
him more than £3,000. But the museum, which was
removed to it in April 1785, had by 1782 cost him
£10,000 in addition to valuable presents, so that it cannot be said that the casket cost more than the jewels

although being on so short a lease it was doubtless expensive. The museum in its new home became continually more celebrated, and was visited by many foreign anatomists of distinction, including Blumenbach, Camper, Scarpa, and Poli. At this period Hunter was at the height of his career; his mind and body were in full vigour; "his hands," says Home, "were capable of performing whatever was suggested by his mind; and his judgment was matured by former experience." There were diverse opinions about his skill as an operator, however; Astley Cooper did not consider him especially dexterous or elegant. Nevertheless his anatomical knowledge and great experience stood him in good stead, and he was almost always successful in completing his operations. It must be recollected, however, that special importance was, in pre-chloroform days, attached to speed, and in this Hunter did not excel. Indeed, to him, operating was a distasteful element in a surgeon's curative efforts. "To perform an operation," he would say, "is to mutilate a patient we cannot cure; it should therefore be considered as an acknowledgment of the imperfection of our art."

The year of greatest success, however, was marked by a period of grave illness, with attacks of violent spasms of the heart, followed by syncope. These recurred on occasions of extra exertion, anxiety of mind, fits of temper, or even the fear lest an animal which he wished to secure might escape before a gun could be brought

to shoot it. To this year (1785) we are indebted for
the celebrated portrait of Hunter by Sir Joshua Reynolds, in the possession of the Royal College of Surgeons.
He was a bad sitter, but Reynolds, dissatisfied with his
progress, one day was gratified by seeing Hunter in
deep reverie, with his head supported by his left hand.
He at once turned his canvas upside down, and began to record that life-like face, which shows Hunter
the philosopher in the true profundity of his nature.
Sharp engraved this portrait, and it was one of his
greatest successes.

The year 1785 was that in which Hunter first tied
the femoral artery in a case of popliteal aneurism, and
thus initiated one of the greatest modern improvements
in surgery, relying upon the enlargement of the smaller
communicating or collateral vessels to make up for the
cessation of circulation through the principal vessel.
This appears to have been suggested to him by an
experiment on the mode of growth of deer's antlers.
Having been granted by the king the privilege of
experimenting with the deer in Richmond Park, he
tied one of the external carotid arteries supplying
(*inter alia*) one of the half-grown antlers. The antler
became cold, but after a week or two Hunter, to his
astonishment, found that it had again become warm and
was growing again. On a *post mortem* examination he
discovered that this continued growth was due to the
enlargement of small branches of the carotid above and
below the wound, to an extent sufficient to restore the

blood-supply in the antler. And by a stroke of genius Hunter saw that a similar process might be expected to occur in cases of aneurism, and supersede the then generally fatal methods of operating by means of amputation, or by directly evacuating the sac of the aneurism. The fourth patient Hunter performed the new operation upon lived for fifty years; a specimen illustrating the case is preserved in the Hunterian Museum.

In 1786, on the death of Middleton, Hunter received the appointment of deputy surgeon-general to the army; becoming in 1790, on the death of Mr. Adair, surgeon-general and inspector of hospitals. In 1786 he published his long-deferred work on the Venereal Disease, which, though printed and sold in his own house, met with a rapid sale, and proved a very valuable work. In the same year he collected a large number of his papers contributed to the Royal Society, together with others not previously published, into a quarto volume entitled, "Observations on certain Parts of the Animal Œconomy," and thus placed his researches in imposing bulk before the general public. The Copley Medal of the Royal Society was awarded to Hunter in 1787 for his discoveries in natural history.

About this time Mr. Hunter was allowed to nominate Home as his assistant at St. George's, and in 1792 Home undertook a further portion of his work, by delivering the surgical lectures, for which purpose he was intrusted with Mr. Hunter's manuscripts. This enabled Mr. Hunter to give more time to the preparation of his great treatise on the Blood, Inflammation, and Gunshot Wounds, which, however, remained to be published by his executors in 1794. Death was about to claim him, and the immediate cause which led to his end was a dispute with his colleagues and the governors of St. George's Hospital about pupils' fees. In his treatment of pupils personally Hunter was always generous, especially when they showed ability and zeal. Thus he gave Carlisle a perpetual ticket to his lectures, having been much pleased with a preparation he brought for his acceptance, showing the internal ear very excellently. He would often also send valuable patients to young men starting in practice, and struggling with pecuniary difficulties. He never concealed from his pupils the hard work he had done to attain his position: "I've been here a great many years, and have worked hard too, and yet I don't know the principles of the art," he remarked to one. He did not, however, get on so well with his fellow-surgeons at the hospital. He so constantly insisted on the importance of studying physiology for the benefit of surgical practice, while they had been educated with little or no physiology, that his manner, as well as his pursuits, procured him the stigma of being an innovator and enthusiast. Early in 1792 one of his colleagues, Charles Hawkins, resigned the surgeoncy, and Keate, then assistant to Gunning, the senior surgeon, was elected his successor by a considerable majority, in opposition to Home, who was, of course, Hunter's candidate.

The acrimony of the contest appears to have led Hunter
to announce his intention of no longer dividing with
them the fees received for the surgeons' pupils, owing, as
he alleged, to his desire that the other surgeons should
pay more attention to their pupils, instead of neglecting
them, as he asserted they did.   His right to do this was
warmly contested, and the question was referred to the
subscribers to the hospital.   Hunter addressed them a
long letter before the day of meeting, in March 1793,
detailing the efforts he had made since his connection
with the hospital to induce his colleagues to improve
the system of instruction, which efforts had proved
ineffectual: one man "did not choose to hazard his
reputation by giving lectures;" another "did not see
where the art could be improved."   Consequently
Hunter had slackened his own efforts, causing a great
falling off in the numbers of students.   The other
surgeons replied that they had continued the usual
plan, and that if students had neglected their hospital
duties to pursue physiological studies, it was not their
fault.   If they had given lectures, copies of them might
have been taken by the pupils and might get abroad.
Mr. Hunter's connection with the Windmill Street
Anatomical School, and his power of conferring posts
in the army, not his superior attention to his pupils,
were the cause of a larger number of pupils entering
under him.   They were able to show that it would be
a manifest disadvantage that only one surgeon should
instruct a pupil and not all four.   The governors

decided against Hunter, for his plan must have produced confusion and discord. A committee drew up rules for the admission and regulation of pupils, and these were adopted without any consultation with Mr. Hunter. One of them, which seemed specially directed against him, forbade the entry of any pupil who had not had previous medical instruction. Young men frequently came up to London from Scotland, recommended to Mr. Hunter, and were entered by him at the hospital without having had any previous medical instruction. A case in point arose in the succeeding autumn. Two young men came up in the usual way, and ignorant of the new rule, Hunter undertook to press for their admission at the next Board meeting, on the 16th October 1793. On the morning of the day he expressed his anxiety to a friend lest some dispute might occur, as he was convinced such an occurrence would be fatal to him. His life, he used to say, " was in the hands of any rascal who chose to annoy and tease him." Leaving home at the usual hour, he forgot, strange to say, to take his list of appointments with him, and Mr. Clift hastened after him with it. Later, arriving at the hospital, he found the Board already assembled, and presented and supported his memorial. During his speech one of his colleagues flatly contradicted him, and Hunter immediately ceased speaking, retired from the table, and, struggling to suppress his passion, hurried into an adjoining room, which he had scarcely reached when, with a deep groan, he fell lifeless into the arms of Dr. Robertson, one of the hospital physicians. Dr. Baillie his nephew, and Home, who was present, made every effort to restore him, but in vain. Thus were cut short at once the meeting of the St. George's Board, and the life of the greatest surgeon they had had. He was buried in a simple manner on October 22d, at St Martin's in the Fields. A *post mortem* examination had shown that his heart was wasted and diseased, and his coronary arteries, mitral valves, and aorta much ossified and diseased, thus justifying Dr. Jenner's diagnosis.

In person Hunter was of about middle height, vigorous and robust, with high shoulders and short neck, strongly marked features, projecting eyebrows, light-coloured eyes, and high cheeks. He always dressed plainly, with his hair curled behind; this had been reddish-yellow in early life, but white latterly.

Mr. Hunter left little but his museum, which he wished the nation to purchase and provide for. After years of effort, in the course of which Mr. Pitt, on being appealed to, replied: "What! buy preparations! why, I have not money enough to purchase gun-powder," Parliament in 1799 voted £15,000 for his museum (it had cost Hunter over £70,000), and its guardianship was offered to the College of Physicians, which declined it, and then to the College of Surgeons, which accepted it, gaining at the same time a new charter and the title of Royal. Hours during which the collection might be open for professional men and others to study, and a keeper to explain the collection, were stipulated for, and at least twenty-four lectures were to be given annually on comparative anatomy and other subjects by members of the college. These are the well-known Hunterian lectures made illustrious by Owen, Huxley, Parker, and Flower. The collection was placed in a temporary habitation in Lincoln's Inn Fields in 1806, and Parliament has granted in all £42,500 at various dates for the building of a suitable museum. The present building, however, has cost very much more than the sum mentioned, the expense being defrayed out of the college revenues for diplomas.

During the weary years of waiting for the government consent to purchase the museum, Hunter's family had to be maintained by the sale of his furniture and library, and his miscellaneous collection of objects of *virtu*, coats of mail, weapons, &c.; and the mere conservation of the museum was a matter of considerable expense. His papers fell into the hands of Mr., afterwards Sir Everard Home, who detained them without publishing them for many years, during which time he himself published a vast variety of papers under his own name in the Philosophical Transactions. It is generally believed that many of these were largely derived from Mr. Hunter's manuscripts; and this the more, that, when at last, after many years of evasion, his co-trustees of the museum pressed him to deliver up the manuscripts as they were, he secretly burnt

almost the whole of them. In fact, Mr. Clift, who became keeper of the museum, and had been long the
assistant and friend of Sir Everard, when questioned
by the Commission on Medical Education, replied that
all his life he had been employed by Sir Everard in
transcribing portions of Mr. Hunter's manuscripts, and
in copying drawings from his portfolios, which Sir
Everard issued to the public as his own. It was in
1823, when Sir Everard had received from the printer
the final proof of his last volume on Comparative
Anatomy, that he disgraced his name for ever by this
great and irreparable destruction. Mr. Clift's list of
what he remembers of the burnt papers fills more than
a page of the memoir of John Hunter prefixed to
vol. x. of Jardine's Naturalists' Library. And the bare
enumeration and contents would give but little idea of
the labour expended in its production. "I have many
times," says Mr. Clift, his assistant and amanuensis
during the last twenty months of his life, "written the
same page at least half a dozen times over, with cor-
rections and transpositions almost without end," so
great was the difficulty Hunter felt in adequately ex-
pressing his ideas. But this only serves to increase
our regret that these valuable originals should have
been destroyed. He generally wrote his first thoughts
or memoranda on all subjects on the slips torn off from
the ends, and the blank pages and envelopes of letters.
He appeared to have no desire of preserving his own
handwriting, but when they had been copied, usually

folded them up, and put them on the chimney-piece
to light the candle with; and the rough or waste copies
on all subjects, when copied out fair, were taken into
his private dissecting-room, as waste paper to dissect
upon.

Sir Everard Home * describes his brother-in-law as
"very warm and impatient, readily provoked, and
when irritated, not easily soothed. His disposition was
candid and free from reserve, even to a fault. He
hated deceit, and was above every kind of artifice; he
detested it in others, and too openly avowed his sentiments. In conversation he spoke too freely, and sometimes harshly of his contemporaries; but if he did not
do justice to their undoubted merit, it arose not from
envy, but from a thorough conviction that surgery was
yet in its infancy, and he himself a novice in his own art;
and his anxiety to have it carried to perfection made
him think meanly and ill of every one whose exertions in this respect did not equal his own." He was
called the Cerberus of the Royal Society, and certainly
it appears easier to admire and estimate him correctly
now than it would have been to live in comfort with
him. Yet, when advanced in practice and honours, he
paid more instead of less attention to those whom he
had known earlier. Mr. Gough, who had charge of a
menagerie in Piccadilly, related that when he called on
Mr. Hunter, if the house was full of patients, and

---

* Life of John Hunter, prefixed to the treatise on the Blood, Inflammation, &c.

carriages waiting at the door, he was always admitted.
"You have no time to spare," said he, "as you live by
it. Most of these can wait, as they have little to do
when they go home." It is certain that Hunter only
valued money as it enabled him to carry on his researches. He introduces a patient to his brother thus:
"He has no money, and you have plenty, so you are
well met;" and he would never take fees from curates,
authors, and artists. With his lack of courtliness and
evident zeal for dissection, it can be no wonder that
his income never reached £1000 before 1774. Yet
afterwards it increased to £5000 for some years, and
had reached to £6000 when he died. But all he could
spare, throughout, went to his museum.

Hunter's sense of his own importance was evident,
and often very ingenuously expressed. "Ah, John
Hunter, what! still hard at work!" said Dr. Garthshore
to him, finding him in the dissecting-room late in life.
"Yes, doctor," replied Hunter, "still hard at work; and
you'll find it difficult to meet with another John
Hunter when I am gone." To Abernethy he said, "I
know I am but a pigmy in knowledge, yet I feel as a
giant when compared with these men." He could not
be described as a good conversationalist, yet his remarks,
slowly brought out, were often wonderfully pointed and
forcible. In politics he was a strenuous Tory, and
"wished all the rascals who were dissatisfied with their
country would be good enough to leave it." He hated
all public ceremony or display, and when begged to go to

Sir Joshua Reynolds's funeral, fairly wished Sir Joshua
and his friends at the d—l.

He was undeviatingly honest, eminently a lover of
truth, humane and generous in disposition, warm and
disinterested as a friend, a kind affectionate husband and
father. Some have called him a materialist or even an
atheist, but he appears to have had no doubt of the
existence of a First Cause. His study of religion was
no doubt limited by natural tendencies in his mind, and
by his habitual concentration on his work, and the evidence of revelation did not make, so far as can be ascertained, a deep impression on his mind. As to death, his
view was, "'tis poor work when it comes to that."

Hunter's remains lay undisturbed in St. Martin's
Church, till on March 28, 1859, they were removed,
mainly through Mr. Frank Buckland's intervention,
to Abbot Islip's Chapel in Westminster Abbey and
deposited in the north aisle of the nave, close to Ben
Jonson's tomb. His name and achievements are
annually commemorated by orations such as those
from which the subsequent extracts are made, but
most of all by the Hunterian Museum and the lectures
delivered in connection therewith.

To expound Hunter's views of life, and the results of
his other philosophical and practical studies, would
lead us far beyond our limits. Life he regarded as a
principle independent of structure; as a great chemist
as a sort of animal fire. "Mere composition of matter,"
he said, "does not give life; for the dead body has all

the composition it ever had. Life is a property we do not understand; we can only see the necessary steps leading towards it." He imagined that life might either be something superadded to matter, or consist in a peculiar arrangement of particles of matter, which being thus disposed acquired the properties of life. As to equivocal generation, he believed—and here he coincides with the best results of modern sciences— that all we could have was negative proofs of its not taking place. As to geological changes, he had strikingly original views, regarding water as the chief agent, and pointing out that the popular view by which the Deluge was supposed to account for finding marine organisms in rocks was untenable. He could discern that in the long past great oscillations of level and climatic variations had taken place. In regard to development and evolution, he had very luminous ideas pointing to modern discoveries. Thus he remarks "if we were to take a series of animals from the more imperfect to the perfect, we should probably find an imperfect animal corresponding with some stage of the most perfect."

We cannot more clearly emphasise the character of Hunter's intellect and work than in the words of two distinguished men of our own time, both eminent pathologists, and qualified as few can be for estimating such a man.

Dr. Moxon * says :—

* *Medical Times and Gazette*, March 3, 1877.

"If we ask what gave him that most valuable power of estimating what was worth doing, and what could be done—the power which Bacon calls the 'mathematics of the mind'—we find the reply, I believe, in these great facts of his history. Firstly, that he was a man who had a free youth, not over-taught, nor over-strained; and, secondly, that in his manhood he worked with an eye to usefulness and duty, and not only to notoriety, nor to the mere cry of 'who will show us something new?' Indeed, the main and distinctive feature of his noble life was his resolute pursuit of the practical aim of his profession, to establish sound laws for scientific surgery and medicine. I have said that the wonderful store of facts he collected constituted answers to questions: Hunter the physiologist answering the questions of Hunter the surgeon. He did not so follow physiology as to turn it away from usefulness. And the results of his work he puts up in his museum. And he will gladly have anything for his collection. But always putting things by in their physiological order, mark, so that in due time they shall answer to his further questions. He will lecture on surgical principles,—true ones they must be, —if he changes them yearly in accordance with his observations. But he will not, he cannot, lecture on comparative anatomy or zoology. Why not? It does not conform enough with his main bent to surgery, to practical aim, to a duty. He believes in a vital principle, therefore he must have an aim before him.

He succeeds in his aim; and by the masterly introduction of the operation on aneurism which bears his name he saves thousands from a painful death. Led further by the same enthusiasm for the true purpose of his life as a surgeon, he inoculates his frame with a loathsome disease that he may have it always by him to study it, regardless of danger and of pain."

Sir James Paget's views * are thus expressed:—

"The range of Hunter's work matched with the time devoted to it. Never before or since—I think I am safe in saying this—was any one a thorough investigator and student in so wide a range of science. He was an enthusiastic naturalist; as a comparative anatomist and physiologist he was unequalled in his time; among the few pathologists he was the best; among the still fewer geologists and students of vegetable physiology, he was one, if not the chief; and he was a great practical surgeon. He was surgeon to a large hospital in London, and for many years held the largest practice in the metropolis. In all these things at one time no one but Hunter ever was eminent and successful. . . . There is not one of them in which he did not make investigations wholly original—not one of them of which he did not enlarge the area very far beyond that which had been covered by his predecessors—not one of them in which he did not leave facts and principles on record which it is impossible to count and very hard to estimate.

* *Medical Times and Gazette*, Feb. 17, 1877.

" In all these characters of Hunter's works we see that which was the dominant character of his mind—massiveness and grandeur of design were indicated in all to which he applied himself. And in perfect harmony with this was the simplicity of his ordinary method of work. It consisted mainly in the orderly accumulation of facts from every source, of every kind, and building them up in the simplest inductions. If he had been an architect, he would have built huge pyramids, and every stone would have borne its own inscription. He knew nothing of logic or the science of thought. He used his mental power as with a natural instinct. He worked with all his might, but without art. I know no instance so striking as in him of the living force which there is in facts when they are stored in a thoughtful mind.

" But Hunter was not only a great observer, he was a very acute one. I think it would be difficult to find in all the masses of facts which he has recorded any one which was either observed or recorded erroneously. If there are errors in his works, they are the errors of reasoning, not of observation. And it may be noted, as a singular example of his accuracy, that when he tells his inferences it is generally with expressions implying that he regarded them as only probable : a fact he tells without conditions ; when he generalises, it is with ' I suspect,' ' I believe,' ' I am disposed to think,' or the like. . . . He seems to have thought he had never reached farther than the nearest approach to truth which was at that time attainable, and that a year or more of investigation would bring him nearer to the truth, and then that which now seemed right would be surpassed or set aside. He used to say to his pupils in his lectures, 'Do not take notes of this; I daresay I shall change it all next year.'"

Abernethy, who knew him well, says: "It is scarcely credible with what pains Mr. Hunter examined the lower kinds of animals," and he quotes Mr. Clift as saying that "he would stand for hours motionless as a statue, except that with a pair of forceps in either hand he was picking asunder the connecting fibres of some structure" that he was examining: . . . "patient and watchful as a prophet, sure that the truth would come: it might be in the unveiling of some new structure, or in the clearing up of some mental cloud; or it might be as in a flash, in which, as with inspiration, intellectual darkness becomes light."

CHAPTER VI.

EDWARD JENNER AND VACCINATION.

MODERN preventive medicine may be said to date from
the introduction of inoculation for smallpox in the
early part of the eighteenth century. It is much more
profitable to dwell on the history of the second step in
this direction, a far greater one, due to the genius of
one man, Edward Jenner, whose Life by Dr. Baron,
though not a biographical masterpiece, is the source of
much valuable information.

The name of Stephen Jenner had been handed down
from generation to generation in Gloucestershire, and
the Rev. Stephen Jenner, father of Edward, was vicar
of Berkeley when his famous son was born, on May 17,
1749. The father, however, died in 1754, and an elder
son, another Stephen Jenner, Fellow of Magdalen
College, Oxford, is credited with some attention to his
education. But his school life was not prolonged, for
about the thirteenth year of his age he commenced
preparation for a medical career by entering upon
apprenticeship to Mr. Daniel Ludlow, a medical practitioner at Sodbury near Bristol, with whom he remained
six years.

Young Edward, when a fine ruddy boy of eight, was, with many others, put under a preparatory process for inoculation for smallpox. This was indeed a formidable proceeding, lasting six weeks. He was first bled, to ascertain whether his blood was "fine;" was then purged repeatedly till the ruddy youth became emaciated and feeble; and all the while was kept on a low diet, and dosed with some drink which was supposed to sweeten the blood. This is appropriately termed a "barbarism of human veterinary practice," but it was followed by exposure to contagion from others in a state of severe disease. By good luck the boy got off with a mild attack; but we may well ascribe to the lowering preparatory treatment he had undergone, that he never could as a child enjoy sleep, and was constantly haunted by imaginary noises. All his life long he was too acutely alive to these impressions and to any sudden jar.

It is perhaps more interesting, it is certainly more important, to notice the influence exerted upon one mind by another, than to examine the influences of any material objects upon human nature. In this light we may view with pleasure the relations which existed between Jenner, his elder brother already mentioned, and the great anatomist, John Hunter. The ties of affection and esteem must have been strong which drew the young doctor from the attractions of London, from constant association with his admired friend in his studies, from opportunities to inquire

such as those afforded by the arrangement of Sir Joseph
Banks's collection made during Captain Cook's celebrated voyage, from prospects of gain and worldly
advancement, to the retirement of a country village,
the isolation and the simplicity of rural existence.
We can hardly overestimate the benefits derived by
the developing mind of the young doctor from his daily
intercourse for two years with such a preceptor as John
Hunter. The impression was mutual, for we find
Hunter years afterwards writing to Jenner, " I do not
know any one I would sooner write to than you: I do
not know anybody I am so much obliged to." A
correspondence full of interest on subjects of natural
history was kept up between them. Hunter's appreciation of his friend's attainments was shown markedly
when he formed the plan of a school of natural history
and human and comparative anatomy, and asked
Jenner to come and be his partner in the undertaking.
Very many particulars of experiments and inquiries
in natural history by Jenner were communicated to
Hunter, and were of essential service to him. His
most important published paper in natural history was
that on the Cuckoo, published in the " Philosophical
Transactions " for 1788.

Jenner's name has been so exclusively connected in
the popular mind with the subject of vaccination, that
his ability as a practitioner and his originality in many
departments of medicine and surgery have been somewhat lost sight of. No doubt this was much aided by

his own modesty; but in the treatment of many diseases his views, founded on the improved anatomy and physiology he had learned from Hunter and his own acute observation, were far in advance of his time.

It was perhaps, however, by his sympathetic qualities of heart that Jenner most of all obtained and maintained the influence which he possessed. He could truly rejoice with those that rejoiced, and weep with those that wept. In him uncommon delicacy of feeling co-existed with a joyous and lively disposition; and his gentlemanly manners made him welcome everywhere. He was ever observant of natural phenomena, and loved nothing better than to persuade some friend to ride with him during his long journeys through the countryside. Those who enjoyed the pleasure have described the vivid and imaginative fervour which characterised his conversation, whether in reference to his own feelings or the beauties of the scenery around, and the captivating simplicity and ingenuity with which he explained phenomena of animal and vegetable life which came under notice. In fact he never met any one without endeavouring to gain or to impart instruction.

Among the many proofs of Jenner's sagacity and acuteness in matters outside medicine should be mentioned the following, recorded by Sir Humphry Davy, showing that Jenner anticipated the late Charles Darwin in his views of the important effects produced by earthworms upon the soil. "He said the earthworms, particularly about the time of the vernal equinox, were much under and along the surface of our moist meadow-lands; and wherever they move, they leave a train of mucus behind them, which becomes manure to the plant. In this respect they act, as the slug does, in furnishing materials for food to the vegetable kingdom; and under the surface, they break the stiff clods in pieces and finally divide the soil."

His appearance and manner in this early portion of his life are thus described by his intimate friend, Edward Gardner: "His height was rather under the middle size, his person was robust, but active and well formed. In his dress he was peculiarly neat, and everything about him showed the man intent and serious, and well prepared to meet the duties of his calling. When I first saw him it was on Frampton Green. I was somewhat his junior in years, and had heard so much of Mr. Jenner of Berkeley that I had no small curiosity to see him. He was dressed in a blue coat and yellow buttons, buckskins, well-polished jockey-boots, with handsome silver spurs, and he carried a smart whip with a silver handle. His hair, after the fashion of the times, was done up in a club, and he wore a broad-brimmed hat. We were introduced on that occasion, and I was delighted and astonished. I was prepared to find an accomplished man, and all the country spoke of him as a skilful surgeon and a great naturalist; but I did not expect to find him so much at home on other matters. I who had been spending my time in cultivating my judgment by abstract study, and smit from my boyhood with the love of song, had sought my amusement in the rosy fields of imagination, was not less surprised than gratified to find that the ancient affinity between Apollo and Esculapius was so well maintained in his person."

So informing and yet witty, so full of life, so true to life was his conversation that the chance of sharing it was eagerly embraced, and his friends rode many miles to accompany him on his way home from their houses, even at midnight. His poetical fancy occasionally vented itself in little pieces of verse, one of which, entitled "Signs of Rain," beginning—

> "The hollow winds begin to blow,"

will probably long prove of interest in children's collections of verse.

Some of his epigrams are very apt, as this on the death of a miser—

> "Tom at last has laid by his old niggardly forms,
> And now gives good dinners ; to whom, pray ? the worms."

Singing and violin and flute playing were favourite amusements of his; and in his later years he would lay aside all cares for a time and sing one of his own ballads with all the mirth and gaiety of his youthful days.

Science and social intercourse were combined in two societies of which Jenner was the soul—one he called the Medico-convivial, which met usually at

Radborough, the other the Convivio-medical, assembling at Alveston.

At the meetings of these societies Jenner would often bring forward the reported prophylactic virtues of cowpox, and earnestly recommend his medical friends to inquire into the matter. All his efforts, however, failed to induce them to take it up ; and the subject became so distasteful to them that they at one time threatened to expel him if he continued to harass them with so unprofitable a subject.

Dr. Jenner did not marry till March 6, 1788, when Miss Catherine Kingscote, a lady belonging to a well-known Gloucestershire family frequently furnishing representatives to Parliament, became his wife. The union was very happy, but Mrs. Jenner's delicate health for many years caused great anxiety and needed constant attention.

In 1792 Jenner became M.D. of St. Andrews, with the view of giving up much of his fatiguing general practice. In 1794, at the age of forty-five, he suffered from a severe attack of typhus fever, which threatened to prove fatal. At this time the experiments in proof of vaccination had not been made, and if he had died, the world in all probability might have waited long for the introduction of this great novelty.

Many who learn that vaccination was made known to the world in 1798, when Jenner was forty-nine years old, do not know that the subject attracted his attention in his youthful days as a country surgeon's apprentice, and that his faculties were ever after engaged upon the matter at every convenient opportunity. He repeatedly mentioned the subject of cowpox to his great teacher, John Hunter, when studying with him in London. Hunter never damped the ardour of a pupil by suggesting doubts or difficulties; but it does not appear that he was specially impressed by what he heard. Yet he made known Jenner's information and opinions both in his lectures and to his friends. But for many years Jenner's ideas were poohpoohed by medical and other authorities whom he met in his country practice. They believed many had had smallpox after cowpox, and that the supposed protective influence of the latter was due to something in the constitution of the individual.

Not till 1780 did Jenner fully disclose to his devoted friend Edward Gardner his hopes and fears about what he felt to be his great life-work. He then described to him the various diseases which attacked milkers when they handled diseased cows, and especially that form which afforded protection against smallpox; and with deep and anxious emotion expressed his hopes of being able to propagate this latter form from one human being to another, so as to bring about the total extinction of smallpox.

The exceeding simplicity of the ultimate discovery makes it difficult for us nowadays to imagine the circumstances under which Jenner had to grope his way in the imperfect twilight, and the perplexities by which he was beset in arriving at true conclusions. Both his own observation and that of other medical men of his acquaintance proved to him that what was commonly called cowpox was not a certain preventive of smallpox. But he ascertained by assiduous inquiry and personal investigation that cows were liable to various kinds of eruptions on their teats, all capable of being communicated to the hands of the milkers; and that such sores when so communicated were all called cowpox. But when he had traced out the nature of these various diseases, and ascertained which of them possessed the protective virtue against smallpox, he was again foiled by learning that in some cases when what he now called the true cowpox broke out among the cattle on a dairy farm, and had been communicated to the milkers, they subsequently had smallpox.

It was this repeated failure to arrive at a perfect result which perhaps gave the stimulus that led Jenner to ultimate triumph. The fact that he was on the scent of a discovery which in some form had a promise of indefinite blessing, made him redouble his efforts when most perplexed. He conceived the idea that the virus of the cowpox itself might undergo changes sufficient to deprive it of its protective power, and yet enable it to communicate a disease to the milker. Thus he at last came on the track of the discovery that it was only in a certain condition of the pustule that the virus was capable of imparting its protective power to the human constitution.

M

Having thus steered his way safely through all the pitfalls which might have destroyed the accuracy of his results, Jenner was able to go on to the next stage, that of putting his theory to the test. It is singular how long he was before he had an opportunity of further experiment. In 1788 he showed a drawing of the cowpox as it occurred in milkers to Sir Everard Home and others in London. Various eminent medical men, Cline, Adams, Haygarth, heard of and discussed the matter, and encouraged Jenner's inquiries. But it was not till May 14, 1796, that he had an opportunity of transferring cowpox from one human being to another. Sarah Nelmes, a dairymaid who had been infected from her master's cows, afforded the matter, and it was inserted by two surperficial incisions into the arms of James Phipps, a healthy boy about eight years old. The cowpox ran an ordinary course with no ill effect, and in July Jenner writes to Gardner: "The boy has since been inoculated for the smallpox, which, as I ventured to predict, produced no effect. I shall now pursue my experiments with redoubled ardour."

Jenner did not, even now that he had attained to certainty in his own mind, rush precipitately into publicity, although his benevolent desires to avert the scourge of smallpox from humanity strongly urged him to do so. Still less did he yield to the temptation to establish himself as a practitioner with a specialty for warding off smallpox, which might have led him speedily to fortune. He was as if forearmed against the stringent requirements which would be made as to the proofs of such a discovery if made gratuitously public. At this time he says : " While the vaccine discovery was progressive, the joy I felt at the prospect before me of being the instrument destined to take away from the world one of its greatest calamities, blended with the fond hope of enjoying independence and domestic peace and happiness, was often so excessive that, in pursuing my favourite subject among the meadows, I have sometimes found myself in a kind of reverie. It is pleasant to me to recollect that these reflections always ended in devout acknowledgments to that Being from whom this and all other mercies flow."

Until the spring of 1798 Jenner had no further opportunity of pursuing his inquiries, for the cowpox disappeared from the neighbouring dairies. At last he had matured his research, and it was ready for publication. Before sending it to the printers it was most carefully scrutinised by a number of friends at Rudhall, near Ross, in Herefordshire, the seat of Mr. Thomas Westfaling. Their sympathy encouraged him and their judgment approved of his work, which none who read Jenner's modest and now classic recital, " An Inquiry into the Causes and Effects of the Variolæ Vaccinæ," bearing date June 21, 1798, can wonder at. Previous to this date, however, Dr. and Mrs. Jenner had been two months in London, experiencing much mortification from the fact that no one in London could be obtained as a patient to be inoculated with cowpox. Dr. Jenner often stated that his patience had been exhausted on that occasion : and it remained for Henry Cline to perform the first successful vaccination in London. Finding that subsequent inoculation with smallpox failed to give his patient any disease, Cline expressed his opinion that this promised to be one of the greatest improvements ever made in medicine ; and he begged Jenner to remove to London, promising him a practice of ten thousand a year. Jenner's sentiments on this matter are characteristically expressed in the following extract : "Shall I, who even in the morning of my days sought the lowly and sequestered paths of life—the valley, and not the mountain; shall I, now my evening is fast approaching, hold myself up as an object for fortune and for fame ? Admitting it as a certainty that I obtain both, what stock should I add to my little fund of happiness ? My fortune, with what flows in from my profession, is sufficient to gratify my wishes; indeed, so limited is my ambition and that of my nearest connexions, that were I precluded from future practice I should be enabled to obtain all I want. And as for fame, what is it ? a gilded butt, for ever pierced with the arrows of malignancy."

The first lady of rank who had her child vaccinated was Lady Frances Morton (afterwards Lady Ducie). The Countess of Berkeley very early pro-

moted Jenner's success and ardently advocated vaccination.

A certain Dr. Woodville, eager to rank among the
vaccinators, discovered cowpox in a dairy in Gray's
Inn Lane, in January 1799, found that the milkers
became infected, and took from them matter with which
he vaccinated a number of persons; but contrary to
Jenner's practice, he proceeded to insert smallpox
matter in their arms on the third and fifth days after
vaccination, as if that could afford a fair trial of the
new method. No wonder that the patients exhibited
pustules like those of smallpox, and this was the first
of the many disasters that arose from the injudicious
zeal of Jenner's first followers. This same Dr. Woodville, in an interview with Jenner in March of the
same year, showed himself so little acquainted with
the real character of cowpox, that he described it as
having been communicated by effluvia; and that the
patient had it in the confluent way. Jenner remarked
on this: "Might not the disease have been the confluent
smallpox communicated by Dr. Woodville, as he is
always full of the infection?"

Notwithstanding the mistakes of injudicious friends
vaccination began to spread in 1799, largely through the
aid of those friends of Jenner who themselves became
inoculators—including many who were not medical
practitioners. In the same year it came into notice on
the continent, the "Inquiry" having become known
in Vienna, Hanover, and Geneva. In particular Dr.

de Carro in Vienna became its most zealous and
judicious advocate, and greatly contributed to the
striking diminution in the ravages of smallpox which
soon became evident in that city through the introduction and wide spread of vaccination. A little later,
vaccine matter was first sent to Berlin. The same
year vaccination became known in the United States,
Professor Waterhouse of Cambridge, Mass., being the
first to appreciate its importance. He as soon as
possible vaccinated his own children, and then had
one of them publicly inoculated with smallpox; and
no infection following, the practice became at once
established in the United States. Some contamination
with smallpox having taken place by injudicious
action as in England, matter was obtained direct from
Jenner, and President Jefferson, with his sons-in-law,
in 1801, set the example of vaccinating in their own
families and those of their neighbours, nearly 200
persons. France and Spain had also followed in the
wake, and almost all Europe was now being vaccinated.

We cannot follow the details of the successful introduction of vaccination as by a triumphal progress
all over the world, proving its efficacy on men of all
colour, of all civilisations, of all climates. Sir Ralph
Abercrombie's expedition to Egypt was the first armed
force submitted to vaccination, and its good effects
were most evident. At Palermo it was not unusual
to see on the mornings of public inoculation at the
hospital a procession of men, women, and children,

conducted through the streets by a priest carrying a cross, on the way to be inoculated. The medical officers of the British navy in 1801 presented Dr. Jenner with a gold medal in honour of his discovery.

Smallpox was still committing great ravages in India and Ceylon, and Jenner exerted himself to the utmost to transmit vaccine matter to the East. The early attempts all failed, some from accident, such as the loss of an East Indiaman at sea, others from inexperience in sending the virus so great a distance, exposed to such vicissitudes of climate. Dr. Jenner proposed to the Secretary of State to send in some ship to India a number of soldiers who had not had smallpox, and to vaccinate them in succession by appointing a skilled surgeon to accompany the vessel; but those in office could not see the wisdom of this plan. Consequently the noble discoverer resolved himself to do what was so needful, and while seeking to defray part of the cost by a public subscription, he headed it with a subscription of a thousand guineas. But before the project could be matured, news arrived of the successful introduction of vaccine matter into Bombay, in consequence of its successive transfer to Constantinople, to Bagdad, to Bussora, and thence by sea to Bombay. The self-denying enthusiasm of Dr. Jenner is, however, as conspicuous as if his expedition had been fitted out as he intended.

The simple narrative which the great man himself gave in 1801 in a pamphlet only extending to eight pages, deserves reproducing in every account of the discovery. Its simplicity is more forceful than any decorative treatment could have rendered it. "My inquiry into the nature of the cowpox commenced upwards of twenty-five years ago. My attention to this singular disease was first excited by observing, that among those whom in the country I was frequently called upon to inoculate, many resisted every effort to give them the smallpox. These patients I found had undergone a disease they called the cowpox, contracted by milking cows affected with a peculiar eruption on their teats. On inquiry, it appeared that it had been known among the dairies time immemorial, and that a vague opinion prevailed that it was a preventive of the smallpox. This opinion I found was comparatively new among them, for all the older families declared they had no such idea in their early days."

. . . . . .

"During the investigation of the casual cowpox, I was struck with the idea that it might be practicable to propagate the disease by inoculation, after the manner of the smallpox, first from the cow, and finally from one human being to another. I anxiously waited some time for an opportunity of putting this theory to the test. At length the period arrived, and the first experiment was made upon a lad of the name of Phipps, in whose arm a little vaccine virus was inserted, taken from the hand of a young woman who had been accidentally infected by a cow. Notwithstanding the resemblance which the pustule, thus excited on the boy's arm, bore to variolous inoculation, yet as the indisposition attending it was barely perceptible, I could scarcely persuade myself the patient was secure from the smallpox. However, on his being inoculated some months afterwards, it proved that he was secure. This case inspired me with confidence; and as soon as I could again furnish myself with virus from the cow, I made an arrangement for a series of inoculations. A number of children were inoculated in succession, one from the other; and after several months had elapsed, they were exposed to the infection of small-pox—some by inoculation, others by variolous effluvia, and some in both ways, but they all resisted it. The result of these trials gradually led me into a wider field of experiment, which I went over not only with great attention, but with painful solicitude."

The great revolution effected by vaccination can scarcely be appreciated in our days, and some testimonies from the past are continually needed. The Rev. Dr. Booker, of Dudley, which in his time contained fourteen thousand inhabitants, testified thus respecting vaccination and its striking effects : " I have, previous to the knowledge of the vaccine inoculation, frequently buried, day after day, several (and once as many as eight) victims of the smallpox. But since the parish has been blessed with this invaluable boon of Divine Providence (cowpock), introduced among us nearly four years ago, only two victims have fallen a prey to

the above ravaging disorder (smallpox). In the surrounding villages, like an insatiable Moloch, it has
lately been devouring vast numbers, where obstinacy
and prejudice have precluded the Jennerian protective
blessing, and not a few of the infected victims have
been brought for interment in our cemeteries; yet,
though thousands have thus fallen beside us, the fatal
pestilence has not hitherto again come nigh our dwelling. The spirit of Jenner hath stood between the
dead and the living, and the plague has been stayed."

Many ladies took up the practice of vaccination with
zeal and skill. Thus, up to November 1805, Miss
Bayley, of Hope, near Manchester, had vaccinated two
thousand six hundred persons, and a female friend of
hers had vaccinated two thousand. Miss Bayley is
related to have carried on her extensive vaccinations
with great judgment and precision. She commenced
by offering five shillings to any one who could produce
an instance of the occurrence of smallpox in any
person vaccinated by her. Out of the whole number
of cases above mentioned, however, only one claim was
made; and on referring to her books, it was found that
a mark had been made against the name, indicating a
suspicion that the vaccination had not been effective.

Dr. Jenner has often been reproached for encourag-
ing unprofessional persons to practise vaccination : but
it should be noted that he never did so unless the
person concerned had carefully studied the subject,
and could be relied on to follow his directions

implicitly. In fact, some of the non-professional vaccinators were more efficient than many professional ones, for these frequently disdained to be instructed by him, and by no means followed the rules he laid down. Thus discredit came to vaccination to a great extent by the mistakes of its professional advocates.

The most extraordinary attacks were made upon vaccination and its promoters, including, of course, most virulent denunciations of its supposed anti-religious tendencies. Opposing doctors detected resemblances to ox-faces, produced in children, as they alleged, by vaccination. A lady complained that since her daughter was vaccinated she coughed like a cow, and had grown hairy all over her body; and in one country district it was stated that vaccination had been discontinued there, because those who had been inoculated in that manner bellowed like bulls.

One mode in which some doctors suffered at the time of the introduction of smallpox is not often remembered. Inoculation with smallpox was largely practised, and some medical men derived a considerable proportion of their income from this branch of their profession. It was stated on good authority that Dr. Woodville, at one time Physician to the Smallpox Hospital, having given up inoculation and largely practised vaccination, his income sank in one year from £1000 to £100; and others who refused to discontinue inoculation and advocate vaccination were more than suspected of interested motives.

The antagonism of vaccination to the so-called designs of Providence was loudly asserted. One Dr. Squirrel on this head maintained that "Providence never intended that the vaccine disease should affect the human race, else why had it not, before this time, visited the inhabitants of the globe ? Notwithstanding this, the vaccine virus has been forced into the blood by the manufacturing hand of man, and supported not by science or reason, but by conjecture and folly only, with a pretence of its exterminating the smallpox from the face of the earth." Again, he denounces "the puerility and the impropriety of such a conduct, viz., of introducing vaccination with a boasted intention not only to supplant, but also to change and alter, and, in short, to prevent the established law of nature. The law of God prohibits the practice; the law of man, and the law of nature, loudly exclaim against it." Inoculation had been just as bitterly denounced as "dangerous," "sinful," "diabolical," in numerous sermons and medical treatises, when it was introduced, less than a century before this..

No more striking evidence of the beneficial results which attended vaccination, even in Jenner's lifetime, could be given than those which attended its introduction into Vienna, where smallpox had prevailed severely for centuries. The average number of persons who died at Vienna in each of the first five years of this century was about 14,600: of these eight hundred and thirty-five died of smallpox in the year 1800.

Vaccination being introduced and extensively adopted, the number of deaths from smallpox fell to one hundred and sixty-four in 1801, to sixty-one in 1802, to twenty-seven in 1803, while in 1804 only two persons died, and these deaths were not occasioned in Vienna, one being that of a boatman's child who caught the disease on the Danube, and the other a child sent to Vienna from a distant part of the empire already infected. Yet so long was the practice of vaccination before it spread to an equal extent in England, that nine hundred and fifty deaths occurred from smallpox in London in the last three months only of 1805.

Wherever he might happen to be, Jenner offered to vaccinate gratuitously all poor persons who applied to him at fixed times. The people of one parish, in the neighbourhood of Cheltenham, held back, while the adjacent parishes accepted the new practice to a large extent. But in one particular year the people of the reluctant parish arrived in large numbers to claim vaccination for their children. On inquiry it appeared that smallpox had been among them, causing many deaths, while those of their neighbours who had been vaccinated escaped. Yet it was not this potent argument which had been most influential, but the fact that the cost of coffins and burial for those who had died of smallpox became alarming to the parish officials, and they were moved to urge the people authoritatively to be vaccinated, and so save the parish expenses.

From this time forward for a number of years Jenner paid annual visits to London, remaining there a great part of the season, incessantly occupied in vaccinating, in giving information and instruction on the subject verbally to many medical men, in writing to a vast number of persons who corresponded with him from all parts of the world, for every one who heard of the discovery and wanted to know more about it applied to the discoverer, and in social intercourse with people of note, whom he never failed to impress by his eloquence and perspicuity. We cannot follow here the many incidents which marked these years, his intercourse with royal personages, the addresses of congratulation and gratitude which he received from all kinds of localities and bodies of people, the foundation of the Royal Jennerian Society, and the like. A few, however, must find a place.

A Dr. Pearson, to whom we shall have to refer again, distinguished himself at first as an ardent vaccinator, but subsequently he seems to have imagined himself entitled to much of the distinction which belonged to Dr. Jenner, and in order to secure this, set about forming a public "vaccine board," in which the chief official status was assigned to himself. He succeeded in obtaining the patronage of the Duke of York and other notable persons. Addressing Jenner on the subject, in December 1799, Pearson says: "It occurs to me that it might not be disagreeable to you to be an extra-corresponding physician. . . . No expense

is to be attached to your situation except a guinea a
year as a subscriber, and indeed I think you ought
to be exempt from that, as you cannot send any
patients." This was pretty well, one might think, to
be addressed to Jenner: in one year after the full
publication of his discovery, he was to be shunted
off as an "extra-corresponding physician." Jenner's
answer showed the sense in which he regarded it.
"It appears to me somewhat extraordinary that an
institution formed upon so large a scale, and that
has for its object the inoculation of the cowpox,
should have been set on foot and almost completely
organized without my receiving the most distant inti-
mation of it. . . For the present I must beg leave to
decline the *honour* intended me." After some discussion, most of the royal and influential personages
who had promised to support Dr. Pearson's institution
withdrew their names from it.

At Brunn in Moravia, where Count Francis de Salm
introduced and widely diffused vaccination, the people
erected a temple dedicated to Jenner, and annually
held a festival on his birthday.

The Dowager Empress of Russia first promoted
vaccination in that empire, gave the name Vaccinoff to
the first child vaccinated, had the child taken to St.
Petersburg in one of her own coaches, placed in the
Foundling Hospital, with a provision settled on her
for life. In 1802 the Empress sent Dr. Jenner a letter
signed with her own hand, with a valuable diamond

ring. In fact in all foreign countries vaccination was
accepted with more enthusiasm than in England. The
proof of this may readily be seen in Dr. Baron's Life of
Jenner.

Meanwhile Jenner had expended a large amount of
money out of his fortune, in visiting London, distribut-
ing information, giving up to a very large extent his
practice at Berkeley, and being by no means recouped
by profits of practice in London. His friends at length,
seeing that he was now debarred from obtaining from
practice an adequate reward for his great discovery, urged
him to apply to Parliament for some reward. This
was at last done in 1802, and the petition was recommended very strongly by the king, and considered by a
committee of the House of Commons. This committee
received evidence which unanimously affirmed the importance and practical value of the discovery, and
almost as unanimously agreed in Jenner's originality.
Admiral Berkeley, chairman of the committee, said
that Jenner's was unquestionably the greatest discovery
ever made for the preservation of the human species.
A grant of £10,000 was proposed on June 2, 1802, and
after a considerable discussion was carried, as against
an amendment proposing to grant £20,000.

It soon appeared, however, that the House of Commons
had failed to satisfy the sense of justice of the mass of
people as well as of the more eminent members of the
medical profession in its grant to Jenner. Sir Gilbert
Blane, in an address he drew up on the subject, said :

" It is the universal voice of this as well as other
nations that the remuneration given to Dr. Jenner is
greatly inadequate to his deserts, and to the magnitude
of the benefit his discovery has conferred on mankind."

In January 1803 was founded the Royal Jennerian
Institution, under royal patronage, and with Jenner as
president, to propagate vaccination in London and elsewhere. This continued its operations for some years
with distinguished success; but Dr. Walker, who had
been appointed resident inoculator, soon began to de-
viate from Jenner's instructions, and to adopt methods
calculated in Jenner's view to bring the practice into
disrepute. Consequently the dismissal of Walker was
called for, but was negatived in one division, to which
Walker had brought in as voters twenty persons who
only paid their subscription on the day of voting. By
such absurd possibilities are the steps of benefactors
to their race frequently beset. The resignation of Dr.
Walker took place soon afterwards, but the Jennerian
Institution did not fully recover from the effects of the
dissension, and on the establishment of the National
Vaccine Institution in 1808 it became practically
extinct.

Will it be credited that, after the decisive parliamentary vote, for more than two years the Treasury delayed
to pay the money, on one pretence and another; and
when at last it was paid, nearly £1000 was deducted on
account of fees. Akin to this, though the amount was
trifling, was a demand made upon Jenner for five

pounds admission fees, when the corporation of Dublin conferred upon him the freedom of that city.

Among the multitude of testimonies of appreciation which Jenner received, not the least interesting is one which proceeded from the chiefs of the "Five Nations" of Canadian Indians, the Mohawks, the Onondagas, the Senecas, the Oneidas, and the Coyongas. Their address to him ran as follows: "Brother! our Father has delivered to us the book you sent to instruct us how to use the discovery which the Great Spirit made to you, whereby the smallpox, that fatal enemy of our tribes, may be driven from the earth. We have deposited your book in the hands of the man of skill whom our Great Father employs to attend us when sick or wounded. We shall not fail to teach our children to speak the name of Jenner; and to thank the Great Spirit for bestowing upon him so much wisdom and so much benevolence. We send with this a belt and string of wampum, in token of our acceptance of your precious gift; and we beseech the Great Spirit to take care of you in this world, and in the land of spirits."

In 1804 one of the most beautiful of the Napoleon series of medals was struck in commemoration of the Emperor's estimate of the value of vaccination. He was so sensible of Jenner's claims, that he allowed his petitions for the liberation of British subjects to prevail. Napoleon was about to reject one petition, but when Josephine uttered the name of Jenner, he paused and exclaimed, "Jenner! ah, we can refuse nothing to that man." Perhaps no more striking example of the extent to which Jenner's influence extended outside England could be given, than the fact that numbers of persons travelled abroad or on shipboard bearing with them, in preference to a passport, a simple certificate signed "Edward Jenner," testifying that the persons were known to him and were travelling in pursuit of health, or science, or other affairs unconnected with war. When the great war was over, and the allied sovereigns visited London, Jenner was introduced, among others, to the Emperor of Russia and the King of Prussia, by their special request.

But in Great Britain there were many things calculated to detract from Jenner's perfect enjoyment. On various occasions the British government were by no means eager to show him a respect and honour equal to that paid to him abroad. When various government officials combined to launch a national vaccine establishment, it was at first stated that Jenner was to be director, with the stipulation that no one was to take any part in the vaccinating department who was not either nominated or approved by him. Yet soon-afterwards, out of eight persons nominated by Jenner, six were rejected. Jenner himself was not admitted a member of the Board, which was composed exclusively of the four censors of the College of Physicians and the master, and two senior wardens of the College of Surgeons. In consequence of this treatment, occurring in 1808, when vaccination was so universally recognised, Dr. Jenner resigned the post of director, but was succeeded by his friend, Mr. Moore, who was thoroughly in his confidence.

A picture of Jenner's inward life at this period, when the subject of a second parliamentary grant was being considered, may here be given from a letter of his :—" As for myself, I bear the fatigues and worries of a public character better by far than those who know the acuteness of my feelings could have antici- pated. Happy should I be to give up my laurels for the repose of retirement, did I not feel it to be my duty to be in the world. I certainly derive the most soothing consolation from my labours, the benefits of which are felt the world over; but less appreciated, perhaps, in this island than in any other part of the civilised world. . . . Cheltenham is much improved since you saw it. It is too gay for me. I still like my rustic haunt, old Berkeley, best ; where we are all going in about a fortnight. Edward is growing tall, and has long looked over my head. Catherine, now eleven years old, is a promising girl ; and Robert, eight years old, is just a chip of the old block."

In July 1806 Lord Henry Petty, who had succeeded Mr. Pitt as Chancellor of the Exchequer, carried a motion in the Commons, that the Royal College of Physicians should be requested to inquire into the progress of vaccine inoculation. The College made an inquiry, giving the fullest scope to the opponents of vaccination, and finally reported that, considering the

number, respectability, disinterestedness, and extensive
experience of its advocates, compared with the feeble
and imperfect testimonies of its few opposers, the
value of the practice seemed established as firmly as
possible. In July 1807 the subject was again debated
in Parliament, and a proposal to grant £10,000 was
rejected in favour of one moved by Mr. Edward Morris
that £20,000 be granted to Dr. Jenner.

The European inhabitants of India were from the
first among the most earnest in recognising Jenner's
merits, and afforded him in many ways practical testimonies of their gratitude. About £4000 were transmitted to him from Calcutta in 1806 and following
years; from Bombay £2000, and from Madras nearly
£1400.

The effects of incessant labours were beginning
seriously to tell on Jenner's health, when in 1810 he
lost his eldest son from consumption, in his 21st year.
This event preyed much on his mind, and left him in
a state occasioning great anxiety to his friends. In
the same year he lost his firm friend the Earl of
Berkeley, and his beloved sister, Mrs. Black. Under
these troubles he felt the more acutely the calumnious
attacks to which he was constantly subjected. Dr.
Parry of Bath, writing to him about this time, says—
" For Heaven's sake, think no more of these wasps, who
hum and buzz about you, and whom your indifference
and silence will freeze into utter oblivion. Let me
again entreat you not to give them one moment's con-

sideration, *opus exegisti œre perennius.* The great
business is accomplished, and the blessing is ready for
those who choose to avail themselves of it; and with
regard to those who reject it, the evil will be on their
own heads."

In 1811 occurred the first well-authenticated case
of smallpox in a boy vaccinated by Jenner, the Hon.
Robert Grosvenor. The disease became severe and
threatened death, when all at once the later stages
were passed through rapidly, and a good recovery was
made. Other vaccinated children in this family were
exposed to the contagion, and did not suffer. There
seemed every reason, as Jenner explained, to ascribe
the failure of protection in the first case to a peculiarity
of constitution which would probably have exposed the
patient to a second attack of smallpox. In fact, Dr.
Jenner had vaccinated the child when in weak health
at a month old. Lady Grosvenor was timid, and
prevailed on him, contrary to his usual practice, to
make one puncture only; and the pustule that resulted
was deranged in its progress by being rubbed by the
nurse. Nevertheless the case created much alarm and
excitement, and greatly exhilarated the anti-vaccinists.
Jenner's simple answer was to admit the fact, alleging
that if ten, fifty, or a hundred such events should occur,
they would be balanced a hundred times over by cases
of second attacks of smallpox. " I have ever considered
the variolous and the vaccine radically and essentially
the same. As the inoculation of the former has been

known to fail in instances so numerous, it would be very extraordinary if the latter should always be exempt from failure. It would tend to invalidate my early doctrine on this point."

A letter of Jenner to Dr. Baron on this subject, exhibits perhaps the utmost degree of irritation that he showed. "The Town is a fool—an idiot," he remarks, "and will continue in this red-hot, hissing-hot state about this affair, till something else starts up to draw aside its attention. I am determined to lock up my brains and think no more *pro bono publico*. . . . It is my intention to collect all the cases I can of smallpox, after supposed security from that disease."

In 1813 the degree of M.D. was voted to Jenner by the University of Oxford. It was expected that the London College of Physicians would have followed suit by admitting him to membership, but they exacted a full examination, which Jenner at his age, and with his reputation, could not be expected to submit to. In the summer of 1814 Jenner visited London for the last time, being presented to the Czar, and having numerous interviews with his sister, the Grand Duchess of Oldenburg. On the 13th September, 1815, Mrs. Jenner died, a calamity which most deeply afflicted Dr. Jenner, and seemed to mark his retirement from active public life. It is much to be regretted that he did not live to complete and publish his own final account, and matured convictions, as to the suitable conditions of vaccination, and the modifications and imperfections to which it was liable. This engaged much of his attention in his later years, but his inquiries were interrupted by illness and by family affliction. His later years were made painful by extreme nervous sensitiveness, and he had several attacks which foreboded death by apoplexy, which ultimately occurred on 26th January, 1823. He was buried at Berkeley, by the side of his wife, on 3d February.

Jenner's nature, says his biographer, was mild, unobtrusive, unambitious; the singleness of his heart and his genuine modesty graced and adorned his splendid reputation. Had those who opposed him known how little of selfishness, vanity, or pride entered into his composition! He made no answer to aspersions.

"All the friends who watched him longest, and have seen most of his mind and of his conduct, with one voice declare that there was a something about him which they never witnessed in any other man. The first things that a stranger would remark were the gentleness, the simplicity, the artlessness of his manner. There was a total absence of all ostentation or display; so much so, that in the ordinary intercourse of society he appeared as a person who had no claims to notice. He was perfectly unreserved, and free from all guile. He carried his heart and his mind so openly, so undisguisedly, that all might read them. You could not converse with him, you could not enter his house nor his study, without seeing what sort of man dwelt there."

"The objects of his studies generally lay scattered around him; and, as he used often to say himself, seemingly in chaotic confusion. Fossils, and other specimens of natural history, anatomical preparations, books, papers, letters—all presented themselves in strange disorder; but every article bore the impress of the genius that presided there. The fossils were marked by small pieces of paper pasted on them, having their names and the places where they were found inscribed in his own plain and distinct hand-writing. . . . He seemed to have no secrets of any kind : and, notwithstanding a long experience with the world, he acted to the last as if all mankind were trustworthy, and free from selfishness as himself. He had a working head, being never idle, and accumulated a great store of original observations. These treasures he imparted most generously and liberally. Indeed, his chief pleasure seemed to be in pouring out the ample riches of his mind to every one who enjoyed his acquaintance. He had often reason to lament this unbounded confidence; but such ungrateful returns neither chilled his ardour nor ruffled his temper."

Such was the man to whom the world was indebted for vaccination; no court or metropolitan physician, no university student, but a country doctor, a man of science and of benevolence, whose name is undying.

CHAPTER VII.

SIR ASTLEY COOPER AND ABERNETHY: THE KNIFE VERSUS REGIMEN.

FEW men have been more renowned in their day than the great " Sir Astley."

ASTLEY COOPER was the grandson of a surgeon at Norwich. His father was a very estimable clergyman in Norfolk; his mother wrote novels of some repute, and was noted for her benevolence and unselfishness. Astley, the fourth son of a numerous family, was born on August 23, 1768. His youth was marked by a succession of hairbreadth escapes and exploits, demanding coolness and audacity. He had no great taste for classics or literature in youth or through life. As a youth he had a handsome and expressive countenance, with much openness of manner and liveliness of conversation, so that he often charmed those who disapproved of his wild freaks. Like John Hunter, he had a free youth, and if unimproved was likewise unspoiled by systematic training.

Both the grandfather and the uncle of Astley Cooper, the latter a lecturer at Guy's, are credited with some share in exciting a surgical bias in the boy's

mind. Visiting the Norwich hospital one day, and
seeing a striking operation, he was strongly impressed
with the utility of surgery. In 1784 a visit from his
uncle, the London surgeon, led to the nephew being
articled to him; but his progress here was limited,
owing to the attraction which a free town-life had for
him at first. One day he was met by his uncle dis-
guised in the uniform of an officer, and the former recognising his nephew, the latter denied all knowledge of
him. The detection of this escapade was soon followed
by his transfer as a pupil from his uncle to Mr. Cline,
who then shared with Abernethy the next honours as a
surgeon to John Hunter. Under Cline, young Cooper
imbibed the spirit of Hunter's teaching from one of his
most enthusiastic pupils: for Cline's judgment about
Hunter was that there seemed no comparison between
his great mind and all who had preceded him.

Sir Astley Cooper at a later period thus depicts his
old master: "Mr. Cline was a man of excellent judgment, of great caution, of accurate knowledge; particularly taciturn abroad, yet open, friendly, and very
conversationable at home. In surgery cool, safe, judicious; in anatomy sufficiently informed. In politics
a Democrat, living in friendship with Horne Tooke. In
morals thoroughly honest; in religion a Deist. A
good husband, son, and father. As a friend sincere,
but not active; as an enemy most inveterate."

Young Cooper was soon actively engaged in dissection, and his adventurous nature found scope in many a

night-expedition with the body-snatchers or resurrectionists in their search for " subjects."

He spent one winter session (1787–8) at Edinburgh,
having already made considerable progress in anatomy
and surgery. He greatly appreciated Cullen, Black, and
Fyfe. Having returned from Edinburgh, he attended
John Hunter and other celebrated lecturers, and in
1789, being only 21, he was appointed demonstrator at
St. Thomas's. Two years later Mr. Cline obtained for
him the joint lectureship with himself in anatomy and
surgery. In December 1791 he married Miss Anne
Cock. The wedding was perfectly quiet owing to the
recent death of the lady's father, and on the evening
of the same day Astley Cooper lectured on surgery with
his usual composure, without any of his pupils becoming aware of his marriage. In June 1792 the young
surgeon and his bride visited Paris, and were there
during the three terrible months which followed.
Cooper spent much time in studying Parisian methods
of surgery and in attending the debates of the National
Assembly. His safety was secured by a democratic
badge, and by friendship with leading revolutionists in
England to whom Cline adhered.

In addition to his income from his hospital lectures,
Mr. Cooper came into possession by his marriage of a
fortune of fourteen thousand pounds, so that he was at
once placed beyond any pecuniary anxiety. He consequently was enable to devote himself mainly to study
and teaching. He went to the hospital before break-

fast to dissect for lecture, and he also demonstrated to students before the lecture-hour. He injected their subjects, lectured from two till half-past three, and three evenings a week lectured on surgery. Further, he persevered in visiting the interesting cases in the hospital and making notes of them. His lectures on surgery, which he was the first in the Borough hospitals to separate from anatomy and physiology, were not at the beginning a conspicuous success. He found that he had been too theoretical, but soon changed his plan, and selected cases in the hospital as the basis of his lectures. From this moment his class increased and became interested. He himself acquired a facility in recalling cases and circumstances illustrative of the disease under consideration which greatly added to the attractiveness of his style. The fact is, he was not the intellectual successor of John Hunter, and could not succeed by similar methods. Yet the influence of Hunter upon him was unmixedly beneficial; he had the wit to perceive that Hunter was not " an imaginative speculator, and any one who believed in him a blockhead and a blacksheep in the profession." The improved lectures on surgery attracted twice as many entries in 1793 as in 1792, and Mr. Cooper was besides selected as lecturer on anatomy at the College of Surgeons. A chief part of his duties in this latter capacity was to lecture on and dissect the bodies of executed criminals. The lectures were most successfully given to crowded audiences. In 1797 the now rising surgeon removed

from his early residence in Jeffries Square, St. Mary
Axe, to 12 St. Mary Axe, long occupied by Mr. Cline,
who now moved westward.   In the next year he had a
severe accident, being thrown from his horse on his
head, and his life was in considerable danger for some
time.   The extent of Mr. Cline's consolatory sympathy,
when Cooper was lamenting the risk to his life because
of its interference with some professional inquiry likely
to be of public benefit, was thus expressed: "Make
yourself quite easy, my friend; the result of your disorder, whether fatal or otherwise, will not be thought
of the least consequence by mankind."

An early pupil, Dr. William Roots, however, gives a
very different account of Cooper's "consequence to
mankind."   "From the period of Astley's appointment
to Guy's until the moment of his latest breath, he was
everything and all to the suffering and afflicted; his
name was a host, but his presence brought confidence
and comfort; and I have often observed that on an
operating day, should anything occur of an untoward
character in the theatre, the moment Astley Cooper
entered, and the instrument was in his hand, every
difficulty was overcome, and safety generally ensued."
No doubt reference is here made to the fact recorded
by Sir Astley himself as follows: "I was always of
opinion that Mr. Cline and I gained more reputation at
the hospitals by assisting our colleagues than by our
own operations, for they were always in scrapes, and
we were obliged to help them out of them."

Mr. Travers, who became Astley Cooper's articled pupil in 1800, says at that time he was the handsomest, most intelligent-looking and finely formed man he ever saw. According to the custom of his time, he wore his hair powdered, with a queue, and had always a glow of colour in his cheeks. In his daily ride he wore a blue coat and yellow buckskin breeches and top-boots. He was remarkably upright, and moved with grace, vigour, and elasticity, and would not unfrequently throw his well-shaped leg upon the table at lecture, to illustrate some injury or operation on the lower extremity. Cheerfulness of temper amounting to vivacity, and a relish for the ludicrous, never deserted him, and his chuckling laugh, scarce smothered while he told his story, his mirthful look and manner, and his punning habit, were well known. His personal habits were very simple; he drank water at dinner, and took two glasses of port after. A good digestion never forsook him; as he said, "he could digest anything but sawdust." He was remarkable for requiring little amusement or company beyond what he found in his professional pursuits; and he read comparatively little medical literature.

It has often been alleged that Astley Cooper was somewhat unfeeling in nature; and it must be admitted that he had not a deep sympathy with bodily pain, for his own insusceptibility was equalled by his physical endurance. Yet he always sympathised deeply with mental suffering, and Mr. Travers, who saw him read a posthumous letter from a favourite pupil who had committed suicide, relates that his utterance was choked with sobs, and he wept as for the loss of an only child.   That his affection was not restricted to his own immediate family is shown by the fact that on the deeply regretted death of his little daughter he adopted into his family a little girl who was no relative, but whose mother died early; and subsequently he himself brought from Yarmouth in the coach, a twenty hours' journey, his little nephew, Astley, then two years old, who subsequently became his successor in the baronetcy.

More widely known than the nephew during Sir Astley's life was his servant, Charles Osbaldeston—a name which in practice softened down into Balderson. He was keenly alive to his master's interest, and had much tact and disposition for manœuvre; he boasted that in twenty-six years he never lost a patient for his master whom it was possible to retain.   Wherever Mr. Cooper was, Charles would start after him, if urgently required, and at any cost of post-horses track him out and bring him triumphantly to the fore.

Mr. Cooper in his earlier years, when anatomy formed a great part of his work, was of necessity largely concerned with the resurrectionists, and was one of the main supporters, it may be equally conceded, of their practices, the details of which he was not unfrequently made acquainted with.   But the state of the law, which almost made it impossible to gain possession of subjects for dissection legally, must be accepted as the apology for much that would now as

then be regarded as shocking. It cannot be strictly ger-
mane to Sir Astley Cooper's life to describe the procedure of the body-snatchers, as Mr. Bransby Cooper has
done ;* but it may be remarked that on occasions when
public notice was threatened, Astley Cooper took prompt
steps to obviate injurious publicity of his name. For a
time the men of ill-fame reigned supreme, exacting
almost what prices they chose. If any demur was made,
they stopped the supplies, and then the medical students
became angry, held indignation meetings, sent deputa-
tions to their teachers, sometimes asserting that their
lecturers were not as active or as liberal as those of
some rival school, and threatening to leave *en masse.*
Thus the lecturers were in a manner forced to pay
more for their subjects than they could receive from
their pupils for dissecting them. Another disagreeable
consequence was, that when the regular " resurrectionists" got into trouble, the surgeons had to make
great exertions in their behalf, and often advanced
large sums to defend them, or to keep them and their
families during imprisonment. Sir Astley Cooper spent
hundreds of pounds in this way. One of his accounts
includes £14, 7s. for half the expenses of going down
and bailing Vaughan at Yarmouth, £13 for Vaughan's
support during twenty-six weeks' imprisonment, £50, 8s.
for four subjects, paid to Murphy, and six guineas
" finishing money" to three men, a douceur at the end
of a session.

* Life of Sir Astley Cooper, i. 334–448.]

The high prices paid led some people to offer their bodies before death; but of course this was illegal. Sir Astley's brief answer to one offer from a third party asking to know the truth, was—" The *truth* is that you deserve to be hanged for making such an unfeeling offer." But under other circumstances, when the obtaining of the corpse of a person who had died after an operation interesting to the surgeon was in question, Sir Astley paid large sums, and was thus enabled to add many valuable specimens of surgical results to his museum. Thus his accounts for 1820 show the following entries in regard to obtaining the body of a man on whom he had operated twenty-four years before: "Coach for two there and back, £3, 12s.; guards and coachmen, 6s.; expenses for two days, £1, 14s. 6d; carriage of subject, and porter, 12s. 6d.; subject, £7, 7s.; total, £13, 12s."

This subject was to be obtained, we read, "cost what it may." It is no wonder, then, that of Sir Astley it might be said that no man knew so much of the habits, the crimes, and the few good qualities of the resurrectionists. He could obtain any subject he pleased, however guarded : and indeed offered to do so. No one could go further than he did before a Committee of the House of Commons, to whom he plainly avowed: "There is no person, let his situation in life be what it may, whom, if I were disposed to dissect, I could not obtain. The law only enhances the price, and does not prevent the exhumation." At last the dreadful disclosures about the practices of "burking" in Edinburgh in 1829 led to the passing of the Anatomy Act, legalising dissection under proper regulations.

Nor were human bodies the only ones laid under contribution by Astley Cooper. When animals were wanted for some physiological illustration or investigation, his man Charles could always procure them, and he had at one time as many as thirty dogs, besides other animals, shut up in the hayloft. Half-a-crown a piece was paid by Charles on receipt of the dogs, however obtained, and no doubt dog-stealing was one source. The menagerie at the Tower was to Mr. Cooper, as it had been to John Hunter, a considerable resource for specimens for dissection. In 1801 an enormous elephant came under his knife, and being too unwieldy to be got into the dissecting-room, it had to be cut up in the courtyard, where, assisted by several students, Mr. Cooper gave himself no rest till all the interesting parts were preserved and deposited in St. Thomas's Museum. Bird-stuffers, fishmongers, and poultry merchants were also among the sources of supply for his unwearying knife.

To Astley Cooper, as to most men who rise to eminence, remunerative practice came but slowly. "My receipt," says he, "for the first year was £5, 5s; the second, £26; the third, £54; the fourth, £96; the fifth, £100; the sixth, £200; the seventh, £400; the eighth, £610; the ninth (the year in which he was appointed surgeon to the hospital), £1100." This was in 1800, when his uncle, William Cooper, resigned the surgeoncy. It might have been supposed that the uncle would favour his nephew's succession in every way possible; but he rather supported Mr. Morris, the strongest competitor. For the rising star made the elder jealous of his brilliancy, and moreover always regarded Cline, at St. Thomas's, as his uncle's superior. Thus Astley Cooper's success was by no means certain, as his political associations with Horne Tooke and Thelwall were strenuously alleged against him. But Astley, ever preferring success to politics, resolved on giving up the latter and on being neutral for the future, at any rate as to all open proceedings. This resolve secured his appointment by Mr. Harrison, the well-known treasurer of Guy's, who with Sir Astley shares the highest credit in the establishment of its medical school. He now absented himself from Mr. Cline's political parties, and always advised young surgeons not to attach themselves to particular parties, as their duties must extend to persons of all views. He also, to leave no stone unturned, personally canvassed each of the seventy-two governors.

In 1800 Astley made his first communication to the Royal Society, on the effects of destruction of the tympanic membrane of the ear. He had found that considerable openings might be made in the membrane without impairing the hearing power. He consequently applied this operation to certain kinds of deafness resulting from disease or obstruction in the Eustachian tube, and in 1801 sent in another paper detailing the results of twenty cases. Although his success in restoring lost hearing was much less than he had anticipated, the operation has since been frequently performed, and the Royal Society in 1802 awarded him the Copley Medal for these papers. In the same year he was elected F.R.S.

Astley Cooper's activities were at this time strongly directed towards the improvement of his profession by intercourse and discussion at societies, of several of which he was the life and soul. The Physical Society at Guy's Hospital afforded his earliest opportunity of this kind, and long retained his active interest. During his short stay at Edinburgh his predominance was so evident that he was chosen president of a society to protect students' rights against usurpations by the professors. Here also he joined a Speculative Society, and read a paper in favour of the Berkeleian theory of matter. One of the debates which he opened was on the subject " Is man a free agent ? " He would have been a president of the Royal Medical Society at Edinburgh had he returned for a second winter, so much did he distinguish himself in debate. At a later period the strength of his association with Edinburgh was attested by his forming the Edinburgh Club in London for former Edinburgh medical students. The most important society, however, with the foundation of which he was connected, was the Royal Medical Chirurgical Society, which originated in a secession from

the Medical Society of London. Dr. Yelloly, who was
intimately connected with the new foundation, says of
Mr. Cooper at this time: " I never saw any one more
open-hearted as a companion, more unreserved in his
remarks, with always a large store of information at
his command, and who was at the same time more
kindly disposed, and abounding in all sorts of material
for the gratification of those with whom he associated.
He was not a reading man; but he contrived to get the
most valuable information of every description, whether
professional or general, and always to use it in the
best, the most attractive, and the readiest way." The
treasurer of the society was Astley Cooper, and he
rendered essential service. The earliest volume of its
Transactions, published in 1809, contained a paper
recording his first operation for the relief of aneurism
of the carotid artery by tying it below the aneurism—
a method now established. But he had previously
published (part 1 in 1804, part 2 in 1807) a work
which largely contributed to his reputation, namely, on
Hernia or Rupture. A second edition was published
in 1827. The anatomical structures concerned were
excellently expounded and illustrated, and the experience gained in frequently and successfully operating in
cases of this disease gave Mr. Cooper a position of the
highest authority. As so often happens to medical
men, his attention was especially called to this disease
from the fact that he had been subject to it from early
life. The anatomical study he undertook in order to

perfect his knowledge of this matter was immense. "I
have related no case," he says, "and given no remark,
for the truth of which I cannot vouch." When his
pupils showed him some interesting appearance in a
dissection, he would say ; "That is the way, sir, to learn
your profession. Look for yourself ; never mind what
other people may say, no opinion or theories can
interfere with information derived from dissection."
The expense of the illustrations to this work was so
great that Mr. Cooper was loser of a thousand pounds
by it when every copy had been sold.

In 1806 Mr. Cooper left St. Mary Axe to occupy
the house in New Broad Street which for nine years
was crowded by his patients, during the most remunerative years of his life. In those years he rose
at six, dissected privately till eight, and from half-past
eight saw large numbers of gratuitous patients. At
breakfast he ate only two well-buttered hot rolls, drank
his tea, cool, at a draught, read his paper a few minutes,
and then was off to his consulting-room, turning round
with a sweet benign smile as he left the room. Patients
crowded his rooms and besieged "Charles," using mani-
fold devices to get the earliest interview possible. At
one o'clock he would scarcely see another patient, even
if the house was full ; but if detained half an hour
later, would fly into a rage, abuse Charles, and jump
into his carriage, leaving Charles to appease the dis-
appointed patients. Sometimes the people in the hall
and ante-room were so importunate that Mr. Cooper

was driven to escape through his stables and into a passage by Bishopsgate Church. At Guy's he was awaited by a crowd of pupils on the steps, and at once went into the wards, addressing the patients with such tenderness of voice and expression that he at once gained their confidence. His few pertinent questions and quick diagnosis were of themselves remarkable, no less than the judicious calm manner in which he enforced the necessity for operations when required. At two the pupils would suddenly leave the ward, run across the street to the old St. Thomas's Hospital, and seat themselves in the anatomical theatre. After the lecture, which was often so crowded that men stood in the gangways and passages near to gain such portions of his lecture as they might fortunately pick up, he went round the dissecting-room, and afterwards left the hospital to visit patients, or to operate privately, returning home at half-past six or seven. Every spare minute in his carriage was occupied with dictating to his assistants notes or remarks on cases or other subjects on which he was engaged. At dinner he ate rapidly and not very elegantly, talking and joking; after dinner he slept for ten minutes at will, and then started to his surgical lecture, if it were a lecture night. In the evening he was usually again on a round of visits till midnight.

Dr. Pettigrew, in his " Medical Portrait Gallery," thus vividly describes the overpowering influence Sir Astley had upon his pupils: " I can never forget the enthu-

siasm with which he entered upon the performance
of any duty calculated to abridge human suffering.
This enthusiasm, by the generosity of his character,
his familiar manner, and the excellence of his temper,
he imparted to all around him; and the extent of
the obligations of the present and of after ages to Sir
Astley Cooper, in thus forming able and spirited
surgeons, can never be accurately estimated. He
was the idol of the Borough School. The pupils
followed him in troops; and, like to Linnæus, who
has been described as proceeding upon his botanical
excursions accompanied by hundreds of students, so
may Sir Astley be depicted traversing the wards of
the hospital with an equal number of pupils, listening
with almost breathless anxiety to catch the observations which fell from his lips. But on the days of
operation this feeling was wound up to the highest
pitch. The sight was altogether deeply interesting;
the large theatre of Guy's crowded to the ceiling—
the profound silence obtained upon his entry—that
person so manly and so truly imposing—and the
awful feeling connected with the occasion—can never
be forgotten by any of his pupils. The elegance of
his operation, without the slightest affectation, all ease,
all kindness to the patients, and equally solicitous that
nothing should be hidden from the observation of the
pupils; rapid in execution, masterly in manner; no
hurry, no disorder, the most trifling minutiæ attended
to, the dressings generally applied by his own hand.

The light and elegant manner in which Sir Astley
employed his various instruments always astonished
me, and I could not refrain from making some remarks
upon it to my late master, Mr. Chandler, one of the
surgeons to St. Thomas's Hospital. I observed to
him, that Sir Astley's operations appeared like the
graceful efforts of an artist in making a drawing.
Mr. C. replied, 'Sir, it is of no consequence what
instrument Mr. Cooper uses, they are all alike to him;
and I verily believe he could operate as easily with
an oyster-knife as the best bit of cutlery in Laundy's
shop.' There was great truth in this observation. Sir
Astley was, at that time, decidedly one of the first
operators of the day, and this must be taken in its
widest sense, for it is intended to include the planning
of the operation, the precision and dexterity in the
mode of its performance, and the readiness with which
all difficulties were met and overcome."

Mr. Cooper, notwithstanding his persevering industry
in dissection, would not have found time to acquire all
the knowledge he did, but for employing several assistants either to dissect the specimens he obtained from
operations or from *post mortem* examinations, or as
artists and modellers, amanuenses, &c. He was very
peremptory in his orders to his assistants to obtain for
him any specimen he required, and would not listen to
suggestions of difficulties.   "So and so must be done,"
he said, and his tone did not admit of the possibility of
failure.   Thus he accumulated the large collection of

morbid specimens which he contributed to St. Thomas's Hospital, at a time when such collections were pooh-poohed, and so little regarded, that he could readily obtain any specimen he desired which was at the disposal of his colleagues. With regard to his proceedings in these matters the utmost secrecy was observed, entrance to his private dissecting-rooms being jealously restricted to himself and his paid assistants. When it was difficult to obtain leave to make a *post mortem* examination in private practice, he would spend a long time in arguing most strenuously upon the matter with the relatives, pointing out the reasons which rendered it desirable in the interests of science. His only child was examined by his express wish by a friend; and he left strict injunctions and directions for the *post mortem* on his own body. In very few cases was his determination ever frustrated.

Astley Cooper reached his zenith in Broad Street. In one year his income reached £21,000; for many years it was £15,000. One merchant prince paid him £600 a year; the story of another, who tossed him a cheque for a thousand guineas in his night-cap, after a successful operation for stone, is well known. Many of his patients wrote a cheque for their fee when they consulted him, and never made it less than five guineas. It is amusing to contrast with his reputation as a surgeon and operator, the extremely limited pharmacopœia to which he trusted. " Give me," he would say, "opium, tartarized antimony, sulphate of magnesia, calomel and bark, and I would ask for little else:" and from five or six formulæ he gave his poorer patients a constant stock of medicine.

Mr. Cooper was appointed Professor of Comparative Anatomy at the Royal College of Surgeons in 1813, being the first appointment after Sir Everard Home retired. He lectured during only two seasons, in 1814 and 1815. Not being deeply read in his subject, he resolved to see what industry could do, and restricted himself to three or four hours' sleep, that he might gain additional time for the dissection of animals. He also employed several assistants to dissect for him, and the result was that his specimens came by coach-loads to each lecture. Mr. Clift remarks of one lecture, "This was an overpowering discourse, and highly perfumed, the preparations being chiefly recent and half-dried and varnished." His lectures were very successful, though he would have preferred lecturing on surgery, which was allotted to Abernethy. In the year last mentioned he resigned the professorship and also moved to New Street, W., hoping thereby to diminish the fatigue occasioned by the numerous visits which he had to pay westward. In the following May he signalised his skill by his celebrated operation of tying the aorta or principal artery of the body, for aneurism, in a case in which life was in the extremest peril. The ease with which he prepared for the operation and the masterly skill and success with which he completed it—without the aid of chloroform, be it remembered—excited admiration throughout the profession, who could best judge of the difficulties which had to be overcome. The patient died of incurable disease, but the success of the operation was undoubted.

After having for some years attended Lord Liverpool, Mr. Cooper was in 1820 called in to George IV., who afterwards insisted on his performing a small operation upon him, although he then held no court appointment. He was very reluctant, fearing erysipelas, and only at length yielded to command. His success in this was followed by the conferment of a baronetcy, which was hailed with acclamation by all his friends both professional and public.

In 1822 Sir Astley first became an Examiner at the College of Surgeons. In this capacity he was very conscientious and considerate, never asking catch-questions, or making abstract inquiries, but invariably dwelling upon practical matters, and putting his questions in simple and straightforward language. In the same year appeared perhaps his most important work, that on Dislocations and Fractures of the Joints, and as was his fixed principle, he published it at a price just sufficient to cover the cost of the letterpress and engravings.

In January 1825 Sir Astley resigned his lectureship at St. Thomas's, owing to the impairment of his health. Mr. Key had previously been delivering part of his surgical course, and his nephew Bransby Cooper had undertaken the anatomical lectures; and Sir Astley was determined to secure their succession to his appointments. He had only resigned in the firm conviction that this was generally agreed upon. His astonishment may be imagined when he learnt that Mr. South had been appointed anatomical lecturer. Sir Astley, desiring to withdraw his resignation, was informed that it was too late. Mr. Harrison, however, the then spirited treasurer of Guy's, came to the rescue, and offered to establish a school of medicine at Guy's, totally independent of St. Thomas's, and to appoint Mr. Key and Mr. Bransby Cooper to the chairs of surgery and anatomy. This was at once agreed to, and a lecture theatre and other premises hastily built during the summer, so that the new school of Guy's was opened in the succeeding October. A large proportion of the old pupils of the united schools of St. Thomas's and Guy's entered at Guy's, and a considerable number of new pupils coming up, the now famous school was prosperously floated. Sir Astley did not lecture much for the new school, though he gave a few occasional lectures on anatomy and surgery, which of course were crowded to excess. He now became consulting surgeon to Guy's, and evidenced his zeal by commencing the formation of a museum like that which he had already deposited at St. Thomas's, and which he would have removed thence had it been in his power. In 1827 he was elected President of the College of Surgeons.

By this time Sir Astley had adopted the habit of

spending as much of his time as possible on his estate at Gadesbridge, near Hemel Hempstead. Here he became a rural character, shooting and "making shoot" with eagerness and joviality. Lady Cooper, having lost her adopted daughter, Mrs. Parmenter, and having had no second child, could not endure living in London. In 1825, Sir Astley took his home-farm upon his hands, and kept it in consummate order, at considerable expense, it must be owned. He was always either experimenting or trying to carry out some new plan he had heard of or observed. He again and again became violently angry, as he grew older, when he found that his ideal farm only produced substantial loss: and used repeatedly to vow he would never allow such passion to overcome him again. One of his experiments in farming was the purchase of lame or ill-fed horses at Smithfield at from five to seven pounds apiece, feeding and doctoring them himself at Gadesbridge, and turning them into much better animals. He sometimes made a good profit in this way, and for years drove in his own carriage horses that had only cost him twelve pounds ten. If they were past cure, he would experiment upon them according to what investigation he might have in progress at the time.

Lady Cooper's death in June 1827 was a heavy blow to Sir Astley, and he was so much affected by it that he resolved to retire altogether from practice. Before the end of the year, however, he found the

ennui of retirement insupportable, and returned to
town and full practice again. He was married a
second time to Miss C. Jones in July 1828. The
same year he was appointed Sergeant-Surgeon to the
King, an appointment in which he was continued at
William IV.'s accession. Having no lectures, he still
dissected, and occupied himself largely with completing his various works for the press. His "Illustrations
of Diseases of the Breast" appeared in 1829, and was
followed by "Diseases of the Testis," 1830, "The
Anatomy of the Thymus Gland," 1832. He was for
a second time President of the Royal College of
Surgeons in 1836.

In his old age, even when travelling about, Sir
Astley never lost his passion for dissecting, and always
visited every hospital and surgeon of note on his
travels. He never liked staying more than a few
days in one place; he soon began to pine after his
accustomed pursuits. On several occasions, when
detained longer than he liked in one place, he would
get up early and leave by coach for London, without giving any warning of his intention.

On a visit which he made to Edinburgh in 1837,
the freedom of the city was conferred upon him and
the honorary LL.D. He had previously been made
D.C.L. of Oxford. He continued his anatomical and
surgical investigations to the last, publishing a splendid
work on the Anatomy of the Breast in 1840, pre-
liminary to a complete account of the diseases to

which it is liable, which was never completed. He died on the 12th of October 1841, in the seventy-third year of his age, at Conduit Street, where he had practised latterly. He was buried, by his own particular request, beneath the chapel of Guy's Hospital. A statue of him, by Baily, was erected, chiefly by the members of the medical profession, in St. Paul's Cathedral, near the southern entrance. An admirable portrait of him by Sir Thomas Lawrence exists. Sir Astley's name is commemorated by the triennial prize essay of three hundred pounds for the best original prize essay on a professional subject, to be adjudicated by the physicians and surgeons of Guy's, who may not themselves compete.

A criticism on Sir Astley during his life accorded to him a great share in establishing pure induction as the only sure means of just diagnosis, and in introducing a simplicity of treatment in accordance with the processes of nature. Before his time, operations were too often frightful alternatives or hazardous compromises; he always made them follow, as it were, in the natural course of treatment; and he succeeded in a great degree in divesting them of their terrors by performing them unostentatiously, confidently, and cheerfully. He stated an opinion and fact to the Committee on Medical Education, which might well have been borne in mind by some examiners since his day: "Whenever a man is too old to study, he is too old to be an examiner; and if I laid my head

P

upon my pillow at night, without having dissected something in the day, I should think I had lost that day." Sir Astley left among his private papers an estimate of himself, written in the third person, which is worth quoting. "Sir Astley Cooper was a good anatomist, but never was a good operator where delicacy was required. He felt too much before he began ever to make a perfect operator. . . . Quickness of perception was his forte, for he saw the nature of disease in an instant, and often gave offence by pouncing at once upon his opinion. The same faculty made his prognosis good. He was a good anatomist of morbid, as well as of natural structure. He had an excellent and useful memory. In judgment he was very inferior to Mr. Cline in all the affairs of life. . . . His imagination was vivid, and always *ready* to run away with him if he did not control it."

"His principle in practice was, never to suffer any who consulted him to quit him without giving them satisfaction on the nature and proper treatment of their case."

Finally, he says, what is a fitting close to this narrative of his career, "My own success depended upon my zeal and industry; but for this I take no credit, as it was given to me from above."

Another pupil of John Hunter, a man of very different mould, in several respects more akin to the master than Sir Astley, now claims our attention.

Unlike many of the great men whose achievements
we have recorded, JOHN ABERNETHY was born in London, in the parish of St. Stephen's, Coleman Street,
on the 3d of April 1764. He was the second son of
John Abernethy, merchant, descended from an Irish-
Scotch family which had furnished more than one
noted man to the Protestant dissenting ministry in
Ireland. While very young he was sent to the Wolver-
hampton Grammar School under Dr. Robertson. Here
he was reputed studious and clever, but was evidently
passionate as well as humorous. The severe discipline
common at that time does not seem to have worked
very well with Abernethy, for he came out of it more
excitable and impatient than he had been previously.
School days were over at fourteen, however, and at
fifteen the youth was apprenticed to Mr., afterwards
Sir Charles, Blicke, his father's neighbour in Mildred's
Court, one of the surgeons to St. Bartholomew's Hospital. His own desire was to enter the legal profession,
in which his fine memory would have rendered him
important service; but his father did not agree with
this choice, and the medical profession was selected.
His master was an empiric; but Abernethy early
determined to get to the bottom of things as far as
possible, and engaged in investigations on his own
account. The bent of his mind towards treatment by
diet is shown by the following statement. "When I
was a boy," he said, "I half ruined myself in buying
oranges and other things, to ascertain the effects of

different kinds of diet in this disease" (of the kidney).

Abernethy's interest in anatomy and surgery was first effectively stimulated by Sir William Blizard, who lectured at the London Hospital, and he warmly acknowledged this in his introductory lecture at the College of Surgeons in 1814, when he succeeded Sir William as professor. He was soon selected to dissect for Sir William's lectures; he derived much benefit from Pott's surgical lectures at St. Batholomew's, and from Dr. Marshall's lectures in Holborn; but was most powerfully influenced by John Hunter, who noted him among his most intelligent pupils. The opportunity of becoming an assistant-surgeon, being reserved to apprentices of the surgeons to St. Bartholomew's, came early to Abernethy, for his master's promotion to the surgeoncy led to his election as assistant-surgeon in July 15, 1787, when only twenty-three years old, by a majority of fifty-three to twenty-nine votes. But he was under the necessity, owing to his senior's remaining so long in office, of continuing as assistant-surgeon for the long period of twenty-eight years.

The young surgeon soon began to put his original powers in evidence by starting as a lecturer. Mr. Pott had for years given a course of lectures on surgery, but no other lectures had been delivered, and the medical school of St. Bartholomew's must be regarded as owing its establishment to Abernethy. To be the life and soul of a new school is enough for any man

in his maturest years; it was more than enough for
Abernethy, beginning at twenty-three, when everything
was new, and precedents were few, and when his own
faculties and studies still lacked much. To this we
must largely attribute the worn-out look which began
to settle upon his face from the age of fifty. He was
not content in his lecturing with any dry and orderly
narration, but combined with his descriptive account
the purposes of a structure, the diseases and accidents
to which it is liable, and illustrations from comparative
anatomy. He for a long time included in his courses
at once anatomy, physiology, pathology, and surgery;
at the same time he kept up his attendance on John
Hunter's lectures, and diligently studied in the wards
of the hospital. His industry at this period was such
that he rose at four, and sometimes went into the
country that he might read with less interruption.
It may seem strange, in connection with the well-
known brusqueness of his manner, to read that he had
an unconquerable shyness in his early years of lecturing, which often made him retire from the theatre to
regain his composure before being able to commence
his lecture. But this shyness is often a concomitant
of real talent and originality before it has found means
to display itself effectively; and brusqueness is in not
a few instances the cloak of timidity. When his
dramatic instincts had led him into his true path, he
soon gained in ease, and his classes increased so rapidly
that in 1790 the governors of St. Bartholomew's resolved

to build him a theatre, which was opened in October 1791.

Abernethy's style in lecturing is described by those who heard him as unique both in communicating his ideas and in interesting his pupils. When his style had fully developed, it was spoken of as " Abernethy at Home." His mode of entering the lecture-room, says Pettigrew, was often irresistibly droll; his hands buried deep in his breeches-pockets, his body bent slouchingly forward, blowing or whistling, his eyes twinkling beneath their arches, and his lower jaw thrown considerably beneath the upper. Then he would cast himself into a chair, swing one of his legs over an arm of it, and commence his lecture in the most *outré* manner. The abruptness, however, never failed to command silence, and rivet attention.

" 'The count was wounded in the arm—the bullet had sunk deep into the flesh—it was, however, extracted —and he is now in a fair way of recovery.' That will do very well for a novel, but it won't do for us, gentlemen: for 'Sir Ralph Abercromby received a ball in the thick part of his thigh, and it buried itself deep, deep: and it got among important parts, and it couldn't be felt; but the surgeons, nothing daunted, groped, and groped, and groped,—and Sir Ralph died.' " Thus he would introduce an admirable discourse on gunshot wounds, reprobating in the strongest language the perilous and painful practice of making prolonged searches for bullets in important organs. He always

illustrated his subject by telling anecdotes, frequently
of a side-splitting character, and so compelled his
pupils to remember his doctrines.

His mental abstraction was not unfrequently manifested strikingly in the lecture-theatre. On one occasion it is related of him that at an introductory lecture
at St. Bartholomew's, when he had been received, as
usual, with great applause, he appeared utterly indifferent to it, but quietly casting his eyes over the assemblage, burst forth in a tone of deep feeling, "God help
you all! what is to become of you!"

His dramatic power was much employed in imitating
his patients' peculiarities, with a mixture of the serious
and the humorous which was most effective. Many
of his stories were most apt in their bearing on some
important fact or principle. One of these we may be
allowed to quote from Macilwain.*

"Ah, there is no saying too much on the importance
of recollecting the course of large arteries; but I will
tell you a case. There was an officer in the navy, and
as brave a fellow as ever stepped, who in a sea-fight
received a severe wound in the shoulder, which opened
his axillary artery. He lost a large quantity of blood,
but the wound was staunched for the moment, and he
was taken below. As he was an officer, the surgeon,
who saw he was wounded severely, was about to attend
to him, before a seaman who had been just brought
down. But the officer, though evidently in great pain

* Memoirs of John Abernethy.

said: 'Attend to that man, sir, if you please, I can
wait.' Well, his turn came; the surgeon made up his
mind that a large artery had been wounded; but as
there was no bleeding, dressed the wound, and went
on with his business. The officer lay very faint and
exhausted for some time, and at length began to rally
again, when the bleeding returned; the surgeon was
immediately called, and not knowing where to find the
artery, or what else to do, told the officer he must
amputate his arm at the shoulder-joint. The officer at
once calmly submitted to the additional but unnecessary suffering; and as the operator proceeded, asked if
it would be long; the surgeon replied that it would
be soon over; the officer rejoined: 'Sir, I thank God
for it!' but he never spake more."

Amidst death-like stillness, Abernethy quietly concluded: "I hope you will never forget the course of the
axillary artery."

It has been, we believe, a somewhat general impression, that Abernethy as a lecturer indulged in tricks
or extraordinary gesticulations. But this is by no
means correct. There was a method in every item of
his procedure, and all he aimed at was to impress upon
the students' minds in the most forcible and abiding
way the ideas he wished to convey. He gained, it is
said, the appearance of perfect ease without the slightest
presumption; and had no offensive tricks. Macilwain,
who was his pupil at his best period, says: "The expression of his countenance was in the highest degree

clear, penetrative, and intellectual; and his long but not neglected powdered hair, which covered both ears, gave altogether a philosophic calmness to his whole expression that was peculiarly pleasing. Then came a sort of little smile, which mantled over the whole face, and lighted it up with something which we cannot define, but which seemed a compound of mirth, archness, and benevolence. . . . There was a sort of running metaphor in his language, which, aided by a certain quaintness of manner, made common things go very amusingly. Muscles which pursued the same course to a certain point, were said to travel sociably together, and then to *part company.* Blood-vessels and nerves had certain habits in their mode of distribution, contrasted in this way; arteries were said to *creep* along the sides of or between muscles: nerves, on the contrary, were represented as penetrating their substance *without ceremony.* . . . He was particularly happy in a kind of cosiness or friendliness of manner which seemed to identify him with his audience; as if we were all about to investigate something interesting *together,* and not as if we were going to be " lectured at " at all. He spoke as if addressing each individual, and his discourse, like a happy portrait, always seemed to be looking you in the face."

In consultation or in ordinary practice, Abernethy was only rough and hasty when something annoyed him. Towards his fellow-practitioners who could give a reason for their opinions or their treatment, he was polite and even deferential. He never recommended interference with judicious plans of cure in order to gain *éclat* for himself, nor unless some important end were to be obtained. He was no party to concealments or deceptions being practised on the friends of patients, and in many cases told the plainest of plain truths to patients themselves. "Pray, Mr. Abernethy, what is a cure for gout ?" was the question of an indolent and luxurious citizen. "Live upon sixpence a day—and earn it," was the cogent reply. He is reported to have been consulted by the Duke of York ; and to have stood before him, as usual, whistling, with his hands in his breeches-pockets. The astonished Duke remonstrated : " I suppose you know who I am." " Suppose I do," replied Abernethy, " what of that ? " And he advised the Duke, in reference to his complaint : " Cut off the supplies, as the Duke of Wellington did in his campaigns, and the enemy will leave the citadel." A barrister came to Mr. Abernethy with a small ulcer on his leg, which had proved difficult to heal. Having heard much of his impatience and peculiar manners, he began to pull down his stocking as soon as he entered his consulting-room. "Holloa ! holloa ! what the devil are you at ? " exclaimed the surgeon. " I don't want to see your leg ; that will do, put it up, put it up." The patient did so, but marked his displeasure by placing only a shilling upon the table when he left. "What is this ? " asked Abernethy. " Oh," replied his patient, " that will do, put it up, put it up," and coolly retired.

It is said that Abernethy's impatience frequently arose from his anxiety to be at his hospital duties; and that instead of representing this in a proper manner, he would sometimes almost push patients from his door. Sir Astley Cooper received many a fee from those who had quitted Abernethy, or would not venture to encounter his rudeness. To his hospital patients, especially those who were in great distress, he was all kindness. Their gratitude was sometimes amusingly demonstrated. Mr. Stowe relates one example of this: "It was on his first going through the wards after a visit to Bath, that, passing up between the rows of beds, with an immense crowd of pupils after him, myself among the rest—the apparition of a poor Irishman, with the scantiest shirt I ever saw, jumping out of bed, and literally throwing himself on his knees at Abernethy's feet, presented itself. For some moments everybody was bewildered; but the poor fellow, with all his country's eloquence, poured out such a torrent of thanks, prayers, and blessings, and made such pantomimic displays of his leg, that we were not long left in doubt. 'That's the leg, yer honnor! Glory be to God! Yer honnor's the boy to do it! May the heavens be your bed! Long life to your honnor! To the divole with the spalpeens that said your honnor would cut it off!' &c. The man had come into the hospital about three months before, with diseased ankle, and it had been at once condemned to amputation. Something, however, induced Abernethy to try what rest and con-

stitutional treatment would do for it, and with the
happiest result. With some difficulty the patient was
got into bed, and Abernethy took the opportunity of
giving us a clinical lecture about diseases and their
constitutional treatment. And now commenced the
fun. Every sentence Abernethy uttered Pat confirmed.
' Thrue, yer honnor, divole a lie in it. His honnor's
the grate dochter entirely ! ' While at the slightest
allusion to his case, off went the bed-clothes, and
up went the leg, as if he were taking aim at the ceiling with it. ' That's it, by gorra ! and a bitther
leg than the villin's that wanted to cut it off ! '
This was soon after I went to London, and I was
much struck with Abernethy's manner in the midst
of the laughter. Stooping down to the patient,
he said with much earnestness : ' I am glad your
leg is doing well ; but never kneel, except to your
Maker.' "

Many are the stories in which Abernethy's name
appears ; many have been exaggerated ; many are
falsely connected with his name. Sometimes he would,
instead of crushing a victim, become sufficiently the
victim himself. A lady once said to him : " I had heard
of your rudeness before, but I did not expect this."
When he handed her his prescription, she asked :
" What am I to do with this ? " The rough reply was,
" Anything you like. Put it in the fire if you please."
The lady took him at his word, laid down her fee,
threw the prescription into the fire, and left the room ;

nor could Abernethy persuade her to receive her fee again, or a fresh prescription. Notwithstanding all stories to his disadvantage, there is no doubt that Abernethy's intentions were most kind, and that he never took a fee from a patient who might possibly be unable to afford it comfortably. For these two reasons, his not unfrequent roughness, and his leniency about fees, he certainly had a much smaller income than he might have secured. Yet his income was very considerable, but not carefully managed. One day calling to pay his wine merchant for a pipe of wine, he threw down a handful of notes, and pieces of paper with fees. On being asked to wait till all were accurately counted, as some of the fees might be more than he thought. "Never mind," said he, "I can't stop; you have them as I took them," and hurried away.

It is now time to refer to some of Abernethy's principal publications. In 1793 he published his first volume of Surgical and Physiological Essays, including his celebrated essay on lumbar abscess, in which he details a simple and beautiful method of cure which has since been largely followed. In the second volume of these essays, a paper on the functions of the skin details some careful experiments upon the air in which the hand or foot had been confined for some time. He detected some carbonic acid in such air, and founded upon the experiments important views as to the necessity of keeping the skin cleansed and in healthy action. The third part of these essays, published in 1797, contained an important paper on injuries of the head, deprecating among other things all unnecessary interference, and so preventing many a fruitless operation. In 1806 appeared Abernethy's Surgical Observations, including an account of the disorders of health in general, and of the digestive organs in particular, which accompany local diseases, and obstruct their cure. Whenever he wished to impress upon a patient or a practitioner the importance of attending to the general health, and the stomach in particular, if some local disease was to be cured, he always referred to his book, so that his phrase "read my book" was expected as a certainty. But it appeared sometimes as if he perceived disorder of the digestive organs in every case. A lady who had an affection outside the knee-joint occasioned by a blow against the edge of a step, went to Mr. Abernethy, and was about to show the affected part, when he rudely exclaimed, "I don't want to see your knee, ma'am! allow me," and pressed his fist with force against her stomach. She of course cried out, and he of course attributed her disorder to her stomach. Nevertheless she recovered without medicine, by strictly local treatment of the knee, under Dr. Pettigrew.

In all Abernethy's writings there was manifested a lack of good arrangement which contrasts strikingly with his excellence as a lecturer: but in the latter capacity his audience was always before him, and he could see and test the suitability of his matter. Education had not furnished him with real literary training, and his aptness of expression and his wit do not appear to striking advantage in his written works.

Abernethy was married on the 9th January 1800 to Miss Anne Threlfall, whom he had met at a house to which he had been professionally called in. His courtship was brief; his proposals were made by letter; he characteristically deprecated too much "dangling," gave the lady a fortnight to consider her reply; and was successful. Not for one day did he interrupt his hospital lectures.

In 1815, after twenty-eight years' tenure of the office of assistant-surgeon, Abernethy became full surgeon on the retirement of his old master, Sir Charles Blicke. He made the appointment the occasion for publishing a pamphlet on the evils attending the prolonged tenure of office by old surgeons. He himself had lectured for twenty-eight years, and been largely influential in filling the hospital with students, from whose hospital fees he received nothing whatever. About the time of his succession to the surgeoncy he took a house at Enfield, to which he resorted on Saturdays, gladly quitting his own house in Bedford Row for a quiet country ride. In the summer he would retire to Enfield on most evenings. This tended very much to the benefit of his fidgety nervous system. From early life his heart had been particularly irritable, causing him frequent suffering. A wound which he accidentally gave himself in dissecting at one time caused him such a severe illness that it was three years before he had recovered from its effects, which appeared in very varied forms. It must be acknowledged, too, that he was not as moderate in eating as he exhorted his patients to be. He frequently was attacked by inflammatory sore-throat, terminating in abscess.

Abernethy resigned his professorship at the College of Surgeons in 1817, and was gratified by a resolution sent to him, thanking him for the distinguished energy and perspicuity which had characterised his lectures. This resignation, however, was not sufficient relief to his overstrained system, which was now often tormented with rheumatism. He took insufficient care of himself, would walk down from Bedford Row to the hospital in knee-breeches and silk stockings when it was raining, without a thought of protecting himself from a drenching. With very cold feet he would stand opposite one of the flue openings in the museum, and this with other imprudences gradually sapped his strength. At the age of sixty, according to the plan he had suggested and strongly advocated, he resigned his appointment as surgeon, but the governors would not accept it. He was persuaded to remain in office some time longer, but finally resigned on July 24, 1827. The succeeding winter was the last in which he lectured, and in 1829 he gave up his examinership at the College of Surgeons. He had now become very lame, thin and old-looking. His eye retained its expressiveness, but showed evidences of the continual pain he suffered. He died on the 20th April 1831, quite worn out, but conscious to the last: he was buried in the parish church of Enfield. Thus early, like John Hunter, died one of his pupils, who, in the words of the Duke of Sussex at the anniversary meeting of the Royal Society in 1831, appears the most completely to have caught the bold and philosophical spirit of his great master.

CHAPTER VIII.

SIR CHARLES BELL AND THE FUNCTIONS OF THE NERVOUS SYSTEM.

IT will have been gathered that scientific medicine and surgery were as yet scarcely in a condition to begin. After the discovery of the circulation of the blood physiological research seemed to halt, waiting on anatomy. It now took an immense and decided leap forward.

CHARLES BELL was descended from a family long settled in Glasgow; but his grandfather becoming a minister of the Scotch Church, settled in Gladsmuir, Haddingtonshire, and died young; and his father, William Bell, born 1704, was a minister of the Scottish Episcopal Church in Edinburgh. Here he suffered from all the persecution inflicted on Episcopalians in Scotland after the Young Pretender's rising in 1745. Episcopal ministers were forbidden to officiate to more than four besides the family; and later, an Act was passed to forbid any one in holy orders to officiate in a house of which he was not the master. William Bell's first wife dying in 1750, leaving no surviving children, he married in 1757 Margaret Morice, granddaughter of Bishop White, who became the mother of Robert Bell, author of the Scotch Law Dictionary; John Bell, the celebrated surgeon; George Joseph Bell, Professor of the Law of Scotland in the University of Edinburgh, and author of the Commentaries on the Law of Scotland; and Sir Charles Bell. The father of these four eminent sons died in 1779, when Charles was but five years old.

The straitened circumstances in which the family were left at the father's death resulted in knitting them closely together in their common struggle. The affection which existed through life between George Joseph Bell and Charles, four years younger, is one of the most delightful on record. Much of the brothers' education was the result of their own efforts. George relates that although his schooling cost but five shillings a quarter, it had to be discontinued when he was eleven years old. Mrs. Bell aided her children with French and drawing, and had a considerable share in bringing forth that talent for drawing which afterwards was of such advantage both to John and Charles.

Although Charles was some time at the High School at Edinburgh, he most emphatically declares that he received no education but from his mother, and the example set him by his brothers, all of whom showed a true independence and self-reliance. He says: "For twenty years of my life I had but one wish—to gratify my mother and to do something to alleviate what I saw her suffer." When she died, the blank and indifference produced in his whole nature were so great, that all ambition seemed to die out of him for a long time.

His brothers made a plaything of him in childhood, but yet appeared confident of his future. They were wont to say : " Oh, never mind, Charlie will do very well. No fear for Charlie." Yet in after life he greatly regretted that his early education was limited, and he took very great pains to improve what was deficient. Even within the last few years of his life he engaged French and Italian masters to read with him, although he could read both languages before he left Edinburgh.

Taking up the study of medicine under the guidance and tuition of his elder brother John, who was already becoming notable as a lecturer, he very rapidly found his true vocation, and gained such proficiency that before he was twenty-one he was able to take part of his brother's lectures. In 1799 he published the first part of his " System of Dissections." Edinburgh, then embittered by the controversy between his brother and Dr. Gregory, and other untoward occurrences, did not give him fair scope for his talents ; and it was decided that Charles should adventure himself in London. This was an enterprise of hardihood at that time, for Scotchmen were still looked upon with suspicion ; yet he had already become known in London by his association with John Bell in the " Human Anatomy," by the first two volumes of his " System of Dissections," and by his engravings of the arteries, brain, and nerves.

The impression made upon him by his first experience of London, on a Sunday in November, was thus expressed : "If this be the season that John Bull selects for cutting his throat, Sunday must be the day, for then London is in all its ugliness, all its naked deformity; the houses are like ruins, the streets deserted." He was soon rather unceremoniously told by a hospital surgeon that they could manufacture their own raw material, and if he had difficulties in Edinburgh, he would have more in London. Some of his early friends in London were cautioned that he was a sharp insinuating young man, who would drive them out of their hospitals. His friend Lynn answered such an innuendo thus : "I liked his brother, and I like himself. He is no humbug. His conversation is open and free." Lynn indeed discerned that a worthy successor of William Hunter was among them.

Charles Bell gained considerable notice by his criticisms on artistic anatomy, and by the profound knowledge of the human body which he made evident. The manuscript of his "Anatomy of Expression" being in a forward state, it was shown to many persons of influence, including Sir Joseph Banks (President of the Royal Society), Benjamin West, Sydney Smith, &c., and the general opinion was that he would make a great name. But Charles did not deceive himself into the idea that his path into situations of importance would be easy. "I can make a few good friends," he says, "but cannot engage the multitude."

After many discouragements, having at one time resolved to return to Edinburgh, Mr. Bell took a house, formerly Speaker Onslow's, in Leicester Street, Leicester Square, and fitted up a lecture-room in it. Here he started as a public lecturer on anatomy and surgery, with an attendance of forty, but only three paying pupils, on January 20, 1806; and the second lecture was delivered to an audience of ten. In February he lectured to a dozen artists, much to their delight. On the 10th February 1806, after nearly fifteen months in London, he received his first fee in consultation.

Many years afterwards, looking back upon this period of severe struggle, he wrote: "When I consider the few introductions I then had—to men who could be of no assistance to me—I look back with a renewal of the despair I then felt. . . These days of unhappiness and suffering tended greatly to fortify me, so that nothing afterwards could come amiss, nothing but death could bring me to a condition of suffering such as I then endured. . . . I could not help regretting the noble fields that were everywhere around me for exertion in my profession, and which I found closed against me." Meanwhile youthful acquaintances in Edinburgh, Horner and Brougham, were getting places in the ministry.

This year his "Anatomy of Expression" was published, and was at once received with high favour, many painters adopting it as their text-book. Flaxman declared he considered Mr. Bell had done more for the arts than any one of that age. Fuseli called it truly valuable.

Charles Bell had more than an ordinary measure of liveliness, good-humour, and geniality. One day he writes: "A band of Pandæans are playing before my window. They make me frisk it. Last night I had a little supper here, with some good flute-playing. It was intended to make Horner know Wilkie, the Scotch Teniers." All through life he retained this sensibility to lively music. The sound of a familiar Scotch air would start him whistling, and laying aside work, he would take his wife by the hand, and make her dance with him through room after room.

By the autumn of 1807, his note as a surgeon had grown, and patients became numerous. His lectures on surgery, too, became an unqualified success, though the number of paying pupils was small. In 1808, however, he had thirty-six pupils. His studies for his lectures were most faithfully and zealously prosecuted. His lectures were most original: his discoveries were given step by step to his class-pupils. The first record of his results in regard to the nervous system is in a letter of 26th November 1807, when he writes: "I have done a more interesting *nova anatomia cerebri humani* than it is possible to conceive." This developed gradually into an introduction to the Nervous System, which was shown to many in manuscript. Meanwhile the Professorship of Anatomy at the Royal Academy was about to become vacant, and Mr. Bell's candidature was warmly advocated by many of the most eminent surgeons and artists. Abernethy desisted from the idea of candidature in his favour. Wilson was dissuaded from competing. Sir Astley Cooper wrote a letter stating that he beyond all comparison merited the post, and would be an invaluable acquisition to the Royal Academy. But in the end, Mr., afterward Sir Anthony, Carlisle was elected, and lectured to but four pupils in his first course. It is to be remembered that even at hospitals, lectures were by no means common things at this time. Several of the most eminent hospital surgeons did not lecture at all, or only lectured occasionally. So that Bell's class of thirty-six was really a first-rate one.

A mark of his original and painstaking mode of making progress was seen in the visit he paid to Haslar Hospital, when the wounded soldiers from Corunna arrived home, in January 1809. The scene was a most striking and impressive one to his feeling nature. "I have stooped," he says, "over hundreds of wretches in the most striking variety of woe and misery, picking out the wounded. Each day as I awake, still I see the long line of sick and lame slowly moving from the beach: it seems to have no end. There is something in the interrupted and very slow motion of these distant objects singularly affecting." From the cases he saw he gained much; and laid the foundation of his essay on Gunshot Wounds, appended to the second edition of his "Operative Surgery."

In 1810 Charles Bell became engaged to his future
wife, Marion Shaw, whose sister Barbara had for some
years been married to his brother George. Their
brothers, John and Alexander, became Charles Bell's
pupils and assistants. In writing to Miss Shaw at one
time Mr. Bell revealed to her much of the sadness and
melancholy of his first years in London, oppressed by
the consciousness of not occupying a position corresponding to his talents, and finding everywhere difficulties. "Many and many a time in the prosecution
of my plans of life have I wished that I were with the
armies, to rid myself of the load of life without discredit." He was married on the 3d of June, 1811.

The next year was another important landmark in
Charles Bell's life. He accepted an offer of partnership with Mr. Wilson in the Great Windmill Street
School of Medicine. His own preparations and drawings, &c., were added to the museum already there,
and his joy at seeing the two united was great and
unmixed. His first lecture in the school was to a class
of 80 to 100 pupils. He was at the height of his
ambition in being connected with the celebrated Windmill Street School. Mr., afterwards Sir Benjamin,
Brodie, Dr. Roget, and Dr. Brande were among his asso-
ciates in lecturing. His new house (34 Soho Square)
had as many resident pupils as he could accommodate; and he was not yet forty years old.

In 1813 he was admitted into the Royal College of
Surgeons. A formal examination being necessary, he

records with amusement that the facetious dogs asked him of what disease he thought Buonaparte would die. In 1814 he was elected by a large majority surgeon to Middlesex Hospital, and immediately began to make great use of his new opportunities. His operations and clinical lectures soon became attended by large numbers of students, and even eminent practitioners. A Russian General, Baron Driesen, having a ball in his thigh, was placed under his care, and especially commended to him by the Czar Alexander. A fee of £200 and two silver cups were his reward, as well as great personal regard from both the General and his aide-de-camp.

When the stirring news of Waterloo arrived in London, the same spirit which had animated him after Corunna, impelled Mr. Bell to start off, accompanied by John Shaw, to render assistance to the wounded. The amount of work was appalling. Nothing was ready, to cope with the mass of misery suddenly accumulated. Mr. Bell, finding after an inspection of the situation that he could do most by taking in hand the needful operations upon the French wounded, commenced his operations at six one morning and continued incessantly operating till seven in the evening, and so on for three consecutive days. While he amputated one man's thigh, there lay at one time thirteen others waiting, all begging to be taken next. "It was a strange thing," he says, "to feel my clothes stiff with blood, and my arms powerless with the exertion of using the knife; and more extraordinary still, to find my mind calm amidst such variety of suffering; but to give one of these objects access to your feelings was to allow yourself to be unmanned for the performance of a duty."

It appears strange that a man who in 1807 had commenced what proved to be such an epoch-making series of discoveries in regard to the nervous system should have so long allowed them to lack general publicity. His manuscript was first shown to his brother and other friends in 1808. But it is to be noted, that when in 1811 he privately circulated a pamphlet under the title of " An Idea of a New Anatomy of the Brain," submitted for the observation of the author's friends, they received it with but scant appreciation, and either failed to regard it as remarkably novel, or considered the views it put forth incredible. At this period, while the brain was believed to be the organ of thought, it was also supposed to discharge some nervous fluid through the spinal cord to the nerves. Little was accurately known about the functions of the nerves: even John Bell and Astley Cooper had advised the section of the facial nerve to cure tic, thus paralysing the muscles of the face instead of relieving the pain. Microscopy had not yet revealed the multitudinous fibres of which nerves are composed, and experimental evidence was confined to comparatively coarse forms. Thus on cutting across the main trunk of a nerve, both sensation and motion were lost in the parts supplied by the nerve. Bell first disentangled the functions of sensation and motion, and found that they were carried on through distinct nerve fibres. He noticed the distinct properties of the nerves of the senses, for instance the fact that a prick of the optic nerve in an operation caused a flash of light to be perceived, not a sensation of pain: when the pricking of certain papillæ of the tongue gave rise to a sensation of taste, not of pain, and when a blow upon the ear occasioned the hearing of noises. Thus he acquired the conception that in the brain the powers of the nerves were distinct and peculiar, and due to the portion of the brain from which they started.

Seeing that in the vast number of the nerves of the body the functions of sensation and motion were evidently combined, Bell imagined that these nerves consisted of different portions tied together, and he sought for a method of determining how they were combined. The separate portions in which the spinal nerves enter the spinal cord, forming two roots, anterior and posterior, occurred to him as furnishing a possibility of experimental inquiry. He now resolved to make crucial experiments on living animals, which should settle the question by a well-devised plan of procedure. No man was more averse to giving unnecessary pain than Charles Bell; no man felt more keenly the sufferings of his patients. The first brief record of the results is as follows: "Experiment 1. I opened the spine and pricked and injured the posterior filaments of the nerves—no motion of the muscles followed. I then touched the anterior division—immediately the parts were convulsed. Experiment 2. I now destroyed the posterior part of the spinal marrow by the point of a needle—no convulsive movement followed. I injured the anterior part, and the animal was convulsed." It was at once inferred that the anterior root of the spinal nerves was motor in its functions, the posterior root sensory.

This simple fact revolutionised the physiology of the whole subject. We cannot now realise the novelty which there was in attaining this extent of knowledge of the nervous system, or how valuable this firm basis was in commencing to unravel the nervous mechanism. We cannot here detail the experiments and trains of reasoning by which it was shown that the fifth cranial nerve was similar in its general plan to the spinal nerves, including distinct sensory and motor portions ; and by which the knowledge of the cranial nerves generally was widely extended. We note now that Bell's first paper on the Nervous System was read before the Royal Society on the 21st July 1821, and was received with great approbation. It soon became generally known throughout Great Britain and on the Continent, being by almost every one acknowledged as strikingly original. The dispute which afterwards arose as to his perfect originality and independence having been so conclusively settled in Mr. Bell's favour by the production of his original pamphlet, manuscript and letters, no account of the controversy need here be given. He himself fully felt the importance of his discoveries: "I have made a greater discovery than ever was made by any one man in anatomy," he says, not vaingloriously, but as a simple perception of the fact.

The application of the new knowledge to the elucidation of many obscure diseases, where the nervous system was affected, engaged Charles Bell's zealous attention. He speedily classified and arranged cases illustrative of the action of the motor and sensory nerves, cases where the muscles of the face were paralysed, as well as various kinds of paralysis throughout the body. Instances of partial or local pain were explained in their relation to the nerves concerned; disorders of the eye, tongue, muscles of respiration, &c., all received new illumination from his researches.

A further discovery was that of the muscular sense, by which we perceive many of the qualities of objects surrounding us, and which even enables us to stand upright. The sensation of the degree of muscular effort put forth in every action, in every resistance, to a large extent builds up our judgments about external objects, and determines our actions; and the recognition of the fact that we perceive this by a sense distinct from touch is due to Bell. The study of the eye entered very largely into this question, as the muscular movements of the eye are of such extreme import in our perceptions. In 1818 he wrote: "I think I have made out that squinting depends on the over-action of one of the oblique muscles, and that it may be cured by an operation. I am looking out for a patient to try this upon." But for want of a squinting monkey to make the first trial upon, the thought was not carried to practical results, and it remained for others to mature the operation for the cure of squinting.

As a specimen of Bell's style in popular writing, to which he devoted great pains, we quote from his Bridgewater Treatise on "The Hand" a passage dealing with the movements of the eye. "On coming into a room, we see the whole side of it at once—the mirror, the pictures, the cornice, the chairs; but we are deceived: being unconscious of the motions of the eye, and that each object is rapidly, but successively, presented to it. It is easy to show that if the eye were steady, vision would be quickly lost; that all these objects, which are distinct and brilliant, are so from the motion of the eye: that they would disappear if it were otherwise. For example, let us fix the eye on one point, a thing difficult to do, owing to the very disposition to motion in the eye: but by repeated attempts we may at length acquire the power of fixing the eye to a point. When we have done so, we shall find that the whole scene becomes more and more obscure, and finally vanishes. Let us fix the eye on the corner of the frame of the principal picture in the room. At first, everything around it is distinct; in a very little time, however, the impression becomes weaker, objects appear dim, and then the eye has an almost incontrollable desire to wander; if this be resisted, the impressions of the figures in the picture first fade : for a time, we see the gilded frame; but this also becomes dim. When we have thus far ascertained the fact, if we change the direction of the eye but ever so little, at once the whole scene will be again perfect before us. These phenomena are consequent upon the retina being subject to exhaustion."

Considering the warmth with which the originality of Charles Bell's views was contested, it is indeed striking to notice how early he composed himself to answer only by silence. "This must be," he says, "the mode in which my opinions shall come to be acknowledged : without some agitation and controversy they would never be propagated. I am satisfied I have a secure ground."

In 1821 Wilson died, and Bell's assumption of the chief responsibility for the Windmill Street School, with heavy pecuniary liabilities, followed. In 1824 he was appointed to the Professorship of Anatomy and Surgery at the Royal College of Surgeons. So he set himself with renewed energy to make his lectures of the utmost value to practising surgeons. His first lecture was given to an audience crowded to suffocation. The crowding continued at subsequent lectures, many being unable to get admission.

On the 19th July 1827 his beloved brother-in-law and assistant, John Shaw, died. His suffering from this loss was intense. In his discoveries, his first great

object had always been "to convince Johnnie." This
faithful brother-in-law was fortunately replaced by
another, Alexander Shaw, afterwards surgeon to the
Middlesex Hospital, notable in after times as a defen-
der of his fame and expounder of his doctrines. In
the same year was matured the project long incubat-
ing, of a new London University (now University
College), in which Charles Bell was to be the head of
the Medical School. He delivered the inaugural lecture, and for some years took an active part in its
organisation. The arrangements, however, which were
made by the governing body were in many respects
inconsistent with the high ideal of teaching which
Charles Bell had, and with the freedom of procedure
to which he had been for so many years accustomed at
the Windmill Street School. Consequently in 1830
he finally retired from the new College, and felt in
some respects stranded, for discovery and teaching
were his very life. Practice was to him an irksome
necessity. Thus a time of life in which practical success might have made him wealthy was characterised
by depression and sadness, principally relieved by a
very unusual recreation for a hard-worked London
practitioner, namely, fly-fishing. He was first attracted
to this sport by spending a day at Panshanger with
his bosom friend, John Richardson. The evident delight
of his friend in this occupation, and the freshness and
relaxation which it afforded, convinced him that he
had found the thing he wanted to sweep from his

mind the cobwebs of professional life. Lady Bell says, "He was often on the waterside before sunrise—indeed, before he could see his flies; and he did enjoy these morning hours. I came down with his breakfast, bringing books and arrangements for passing the whole day, even with cloaks and umbrellas, for no weather deterred us. He liked me to see him land his fish, and waved his hat for me to come." In the intervals of angling many of the best parts of his popular works on the Hand and on Animal Mechanics were written.

In spite of the feelings of disappointment which oppressed him severely on some occasions, it must not be imagined that he was predominantly unhappy. Lord Jeffrey described him as "happy Charlie Bell;" Lord Cockburn wrote: "If I ever knew a generally and practically happy man, it was Sir Charles Bell." Alexander Shaw said of him: "His mind was a garden of flowers and a forest of hardy trees. Its exercise in profound thought gave him high enjoyment; yet he would often avow his pleasure in being still a boy, and he did love life and nature with the freshness of youth. I therefore repeat—if ever I knew a happy man, it was Sir Charles Bell." Yet, seeing that he was convinced, "that the place of a professor who *fills his place* is the most respectable in life," we may believe that a painful sense of ungratified desire was largely present if not continually expressed. In 1835 he writes: "My hands are better for operation than any I have seen at work; but an operating surgeon's life has no equivalent reward in this world .. I must be the teacher and consulting surgeon to be happy."

In 1831, in connection with the accession of William IV., the Guelphic order of knighthood was conferred on several distinguished men of science, among whom Charles Bell was included. His association with Herschel and Brewster in this honour was gratifying and appropriate. A complete school of medicine was now projected in connection with the Middlesex Hospital, in which he was to take a prominent part. It had not, however, passed through three complete months of its history, when the Town Council of Edinburgh elected Sir Charles * to the Chair of Surgery in the University, and the offer proved attractive enough to induce him to leave London. He had always cherished the idea of a return to Edinburgh at some future time, and it appeared to him that there was a possibility of a sphere of more elevated usefulness there, than he could now hope for in London. Moreover, his heart was in Scotland, in the streets of Edinburgh—in the theatre where Monro had lectured to him—in the society of his old friends Jeffrey, Cockburn, William Clerk, Adam Ferguson, and most of all his brother George. "London is a place to live in, but not to die in," he said. "My comfort has ever been to labour for some great purpose, and my great object of study has been attained . . . There is but one place where I can hope to fulfil the object

* In December 1835.

of my scientific labour, and that is Edinburgh; and that is an experiment."

Successful as his classes were in Edinburgh, and influential as his position speedily became, it must be acknowledged that the experiment was a failure, for it did not give him the satisfaction he had hoped. Practice in Edinburgh could not possibly yield what London did, and the emoluments of the University chair did not counterbalance this. Some coldness, too, was shown him on the part of his fellow-professors. It was an old case of Scotch undemonstrativeness. "I have had a German professor to breakfast," he writes, "who brings me a volume from Paris—they make me greater than Harvey. I wish to heaven the folks at home would make something of me. I thought, in addressing the new-made doctors at the conclusion of the session, that I had done well; but not one word of approbation from any professor, nor has one of them in all this time called me in to consultation, except when forced by the desire of the patient." His income, never very considerable in Edinburgh, diminished considerably. "I put down my carriage with as little feeling as I throw off my shoes," he says; but when in 1842 a Government proposal appeared likely to end in the extinction of the privileges of his beloved University, his excitement was unbounded. He set off for London as soon as he could. But he was attacked by a spasm of the stomach so severe as to threaten his life. He hastened

on towards London, but while at Manchester, assisting
at an operation, he thought he should have been obliged
to lie and roll on the carpet, or leave the room in
the midst of it. On Wednesday April 27, 1842, Sir
Charles and Lady Bell reached Hallow Park, the
seat of Mrs. Holland, near Worcester. Looking on
the winding Severn and the distant hills, he said to
his wife: "This is a novel spot; here I fain would
rest till they come to take me away." Here he
sketched an old yew-tree, some sheep, and the river;
then two children and a donkey. As he went back
he looked with his observant eye at every shrub,
commented on the birds' notes, and gathered up their
feathers for his flies. After dinner the same evening
he gave graphic sketches of medical celebrities he
had known, admired and discussed an engraving of
Leonardo da Vinci's Last Supper, and was altogether
so happy in mood that he said to his wife: "Did you
ever see me happier or better than I have been all
this forenoon?" yet he had been several times that
day in imminent danger of death from the dread
malady that John Hunter had, angina pectoris. We
cannot refrain from quoting the account of his end
(Letters, p. 400): "The evening reading that night
was the 23d Psalm; the last prayer, that beautiful
one, 'For that peace which the world cannot give,'
and then he sank into a deep and quiet sleep. In
the morning he awoke with a spasm, which he said
was caused by changing his position. His wife was

rising to drop his laudanum for him, but calling her to him, he laid his head on her shoulder, and there 'rested.'"

No more appropriate tribute has been paid to Sir Charles Bell than that in the *Edinburgh Review* for April 1872. The writer says (p. 429): "Never passed away a gentler, truer, or finer spirit. His genius was great, and has left a legacy to mankind which will keep his name fresh in many generations. But the story of his life has a more potent moral. It is the story of one who kept his affections young, and his love of the pure and the refined unsullied, while fighting bravely the battle of life; whose heart was as tender as his intellect was vigorous and original who, while he gained a foremost place among his fellows, turned with undiminished zest to his home and his friends, and found there the object, the reward, and the solace of his life."

He was buried near the yew-tree he had so lately sketched in Hallow Churchyard. A plain stone, with his name, dates of birth and death, and the line, "The pure in heart shall see God," marked the spot. A tablet was afterwards placed in the churchyard, with an inscription written by his lifelong friend Francis (Lord) Jeffrey. Part of it runs thus: "Sacred to the memory of Sir Charles Bell, who, after unfolding with unrivalled sagacity, patience, and success, the wonderful structure of our mortal bodies, esteemed lightly of his greatest discoveries, except only as they tended to impress himself and others with a deeper sense of the infinite wisdom and ineffable goodness of the Almighty Creator." His letters, edited by his widow (1870), are a lasting memorial of his beautiful and noble nature.

CHAPTER IX.

MARSHALL HALL, AND THE DISCOVERY OF REFLEX ACTION.

THE character of MARSHALL HALL, who divides with Sir Charles Bell the principal honours of discovery as to the nervous system, presents a contrast to his in that it displays a mind more minutely active, and more distinctly medical in its tone, combined with a marvellous degree of detailed benevolence. Thus Hall's reputation has, like Harvey's and John Hunter's, grown largely since his death. Marshall Hall was born at Basford near Nottingham on February 18, 1790, his father, Robert Hall, having been a cotton manufacturer and bleacher of ingenuity and originality. He first employed chlorine as a bleaching agent on a large scale, his earliest attempts having procured for his establishment the epithet of "Bedlam." He was of a very religious turn, too, being one of the early Wesleyans. The strict but benevolent piety of his father, and the sweet and gentle disposition of his mother, were favourable to the growth of high morality, strict conscientiousness, and amiability of character in their family, while the inventive ability of the father reproduced itself in his second son, Samuel Hall, a prolific inventor, and no less in his sixth son, Marshall. It is not often that a typically good and inoffensive son has turned out so conspicuously original in his work. But he had a saving fondness for boyish literature such as Robinson Crusoe, and was full of fun and playfulness. He was early sent to Nottingham to school with the Rev. J. Blanchard, the instructor of Kirke White. Here he did not even learn Latin, although his elder brothers had had classical instruction. French appears to have been his only linguistic attainment : and the chief fact recorded of his school-days is his thrashing a tyrannical "big boy" in the school. But school was over for him at the age of 14, and he was placed with a chemist at Newark. Soon finding his position irksome, his friendship with a youth who was preparing for a medical career led him to long for a similar course, and ultimately his father was induced to send him to Edinburgh, whither he went in October 1809. He had already indicated his future eminence by rising very early to study medicine and chemistry, and giving as his reason: "I am determined to be a great man."

At Edinburgh he quickly distinguished himself by his diligent study of anatomy ; he was recognised as a student of the first rank, and was chosen senior president of the Royal Medical Society in 1811. Dr. Bigsby says of him: "Few men have changed during

their progress through life so little as Marshall Hall.
As he began, so he ended, delighting in the labour—the
labour itself—of investigation. . . . All the stores of
knowledge which his predecessors had either gathered
or created, Marshall Hall was eager to acquire; a hardy,
enduring constitution seconding all his efforts. . . . All
his energies were directed to the formation of the skilful
bedside physician, that is, to the alleviation and cure
of disease." It was said of him, "Hall never tires."
During his three years' studentship he never once
missed a lecture. He graduated in June 1812, and
was almost at once appointed resident house physician
to the Edinburgh Royal Infirmary. Here his love of
order, his zeal, and spirit of inquiry found full scope, and
he took extreme pains in the study of diagnosis. He
gave a voluntary course of lectures on the principles of
diagnosis in 1813, which were the basis of his well-
known work, first published in 1817. His usefulness
to the younger students in the hospital was very great,
and equally striking was his good example of purity of
life and conversation, and constant cheerfulness. His
puremindedness was characteristic through life; Marshall Hall never attached himself to any man of coarse
mind or manners.

During his last year at Edinburgh the young
physician, attracted towards London practice, was
prudently weighing the cost and risk of such an enterprise. He decided in favour of a more modest course
of provincial practice, waiting till his book on Diagnosis

should be matured. As in later life, so now he was "strong in hope, inflexible for truth and justice, but inexperienced in the ways of the world, and unable to cope with the cunning, or to dissemble with the false." After a visit to Paris for some months he proceeded to Göttingen and on to Berlin to visit the medical schools, walking alone and on foot from Paris to Göttingen, more than six hundred miles, in November 1814. After a brief period of practice in Bridgewater he commenced practice at Nottingham in February 1817, and with remarkable rapidity attained a leading position. In 1817 his work on the Diagnosis of Diseases appeared, and at once marked him out as a man of the highest originality, applying accurate observation and classification of symptoms to the detection and distinction of diseases. Of this book the *Lancet* of August 15, 1857, remarked: "Comprehensive, lucid, exact, and reliable, this work has, in the main, stood the test of forty years' trial. A better has not been produced." When Dr. Baillie, nephew of John Hunter and President of the College of Physicians, first saw Marshall Hall, he complimented him on being the son of the author of so extraordinary a work as that on Diagnosis. Being modestly told that he himself was the author, Baillie exclaimed: "Impossible! it would have done credit to the greyest-headed philosopher in our profession."

In 1818 Hall published a work on the affections usually denominated Bilious, Nervous, &c., and in 1820 an essay in which the prevalent custom of bleeding was attacked, especially in certain affections occurring after childbirth, which under that treatment almost invariably proved fatal. In 1822 this was followed by a small volume on the Symptoms and History of Diseases, which was especially valuable in treating of the detection of internal diseases. In 1824 appeared his important paper On the Effects of the Loss of Blood in the "Medico-Chirurgical Transactions," published also in an expanded form in his "Medical Essays" in the same year. Before this time the lancet was in hourly use, and Marshall Hall termed it "a minute instrument of mighty mischief." Almost all pain in any complaint, quickness of pulse, headache, intolerance of light or noise, being believed to arise from inflammation, blood flowed in torrents to subdue it. It was by his various papers bearing on this question that Dr. Hall became prominently known; for the dropping of the lancet was an evident change of procedure which the public as well as the profession could lay hold of. In 1825 the young enemy of the lancet was elected Physician to the Nottingham Hospital by a large majority of votes, and the best practice of the neighbouring counties was his. He was unremittingly employed: in his walks and rides almost heedless of external occurrences, absorbed in contemplation; at home ever busy in his library or his laboratory, making chemical experiments from which numerous valuable memoirs arose; never accepting invitations of pleasure; unwearied in his attentions to the sick poor whom he saw gratuitously. He economised time by riding, being a good horseman, riding through the country on pitch-dark nights without accidents. He treated his horses well and earned their affection. " How is it that your horses never fall?" a friend inquired. "I never give them time to fall," was the reply. The Bible constantly at his side was another mark of Marshall Hall, and he was ever ready to discourse on the wisdom and benevolence of God, as shown in the structure of the human body.

London continued to attract the popular Nottingham physician. Dr. Baillie had predicted that if he came to London, he would be the leading physician in five years; Sir Henry Halford, who succeeded him as President of the College of Physicians, termed Marshall Hall, a few years afterwards, "the rising sun of the profession." We cannot wonder that a visit to London in August 1826 resulted in his remaining there. His Nottingham patients, deeply regretting his removal, continued to consult him by letter; and his first year in town produced £800, a remarkable instance of quick success.

In 1828 he published " Commentaries on Diseases of Females," with graphic plates depicting conditions of parts such as the tongue, lips, nails, &c., which he first associated with various disorders of women. He continued his series of careful papers on subjects connected with blood-letting. His writings on these two subjects produced him a considerable portion of his early practice.

Meantime Marshall Hall married, in 1829, and soon afterwards settled in Manchester Square, where he lived for twenty years. Desiring to become a Fellow of the Royal Society, he entered upon a special research on the circulation of the blood, the results of which he might communicate to the Society. After carefully inspecting under the microscope the blood-flow in the transparent parts of frogs, toads, newts, &c., he arrived at the conclusion that all the blood changes, and all nutrition and absorption by the material tissues are effected in the minute or capillary channels between the arteries and the veins. The paper founded upon this research was read before the Royal Society in 1831, but was refused a place in the "Philosophical Transactions;" yet an equally great man, Johannes Müller, the leading German physiologist, pronounced his paper one of extraordinary interest. It was separately published in 1832. The Royal Society, however, did not reject Marshall Hall's next paper, "On the Inverse Ratio between Respiration and Irritability in the Animal Kingdom," which has been pronounced "one of the most beautiful examples of widely extended observations, and previously disjointed facts, all brought together and rendered harmonious by the insight and genius of a master-mind." *

From the latter subject the investigator passed to that of hybernation, his views on which also found acceptance with the Royal Society. One feature in

* *Medical Times and Gazette* August 29, 1857.

his experiments on this subject was an ingenious apparatus for ascertaining the temperature of the bat without disturbing its winter sleep. By this time Marshall Hall had quite a little menagerie in his house, of animals whose physiology he was investigating; mice, hedgehogs, bats, birds, snakes, frogs, toads, newts, fishes were in turn laid under contribution. Abhorring cruelty as utterly as a man could, he yet saw the absolute necessity of discovering in the first instance, by experiments on animals, truths which were of vital importance both to men and brutes. Mr. Henry Smith of Torrington Square was his diligent associate in these inquiries. Dr. Hall said of him: "I never knew a person so accurate in his information and so devoid of selfishness. His interest in my researches never flagged. He was true to his appointments as the clock itself."

While the papers refused a place in the "Philosophical Transactions" were going through the press, to appear as a "Critical and Experimental Essay on the Circulation of the Blood," a serious accident happened to a portion of the manuscript. It was sent from time to time by stage-coach to Messrs. Seeley, printers, at Thames Ditton, and on the evening of William IV.'s coronation a packet containing the only record of a considerable series of experiments was stolen from the coach. This most serious loss could only be repaired by a repetition of the experiments, which Dr. Hall at once set about with most Christian equanimity.

Early in 1832 Marshall Hall was elected a Fellow of

the Royal Society, and in the same year he published another paper on the Effects of Loss of Blood, in the "Medico-Chirurgical Transactions." The original papers on practical medicine which he produced during this period are too numerous to be mentioned here. We must hasten to give an account of Marshall Hall's great researches on the reflex functions of the spinal cord.

It was while he was examining the circulation of the blood in the newt's lung that Marshall Hall noted the fact from which his great discoveries arose. The newt's head had been cut off; thus its life, in the ordinary acceptation, was destroyed. The tail was afterwards separated. "I now touched the external integument with the point of a needle; it moved with energy, assuming various curvilinear forms! What was the nature of this phenomenon? I had not touched a muscle; I had not touched a muscular nerve; I had not touched the spinal marrow. I had touched a cutaneous nerve. That the influence of this touch was exerted through the spinal marrow was demonstrated by the fact that the phenomenon ceased when the spinal marrow was destroyed. It was obvious that the same influence was reflected along the muscular nerve to the muscles, for the phenomenon again ceased when these nerves were divided. And thus we had the most perfect evidence of a reflex, or diastaltic, or diacentric action."

The importance of this discovery may be gathered from the fact, that but few considerable advances in the physiology of the nervous system had hitherto been made, the most important being that of Sir Charles Bell, proving that there were separate nerve-fibres of motion and of sensation, and that they entered different portions of the spinal cord and brain. Dr. Andrew Whytt of Edinburgh had published in 1751 a work in which he detailed the movements which a frog's trunk was able to execute after its head had been cut off, and had naturally referred these movements to the spinal cord; but the import of such actions was not understood, nor the mechanism by which they were executed. Somehow these observations led to no new principles. But the truly original mind of Marshall Hall travelled beyond the first facts to trace the process, and he at last comprehended the nature of such acts as the involuntary closure of the eyelids, independent of will, for the purpose of preventing the admission of injurious matter, or of protecting the eye against injury. The processes of swallowing, choking, vomiting, coughing were now for the first time explained. Further, in pursuance of Marshall Hall's practicality of object, many cases of injury to the nervous system became more or less intelligible. In paralysis of the brain, where the medulla oblongata and spinal cord were uninjured, it was understood how the animal functions could be maintained, and how in cases where the patient was unable by any exercise of the will to clench his hand, yet the stimulus of a rough stick on the sensory nerves of the palm of the hand was sufficient to bring about a forcible grasp, this being a simple reflex act in which the spinal cord was concerned. The first breath of a new-born infant, the spasmodic closure of the larynx in convulsions, fits of spasmodic asthma, &c., were seen to be reflex in their nature; and in many disorders which had hitherto baffled curative efforts, they became possible, because the first great step had been taken, the understanding of the phenomena.

These discoveries proved so far-reaching in their bearing that their establishment and following out were the work of years of almost constant toil. It is estimated that from the period of his first experiments to the close of his life no fewer than thirty-five thousand hours were occupied by Dr. Hall in work strictly connected with the subject. The discovery was first made known to the Zoological Society on November 27, 1832: a fuller and further account was given to the Royal Society in 1833, and published in the Transactions. It was immediately translated into German and inserted in Müller's Archiv. Yet most of the leading authorities in England, with the fatality which attends discoveries in proportion to their greatness, made Marshall Hall the object of obloquy, and denounced him as the propagator of absurd and idle theories. In 1837 a second memoir was read before the Royal Society, but was rejected from its Transactions; and in a most unscientific spirit, Dr. Hall's offer to show his experiments before a committee was not acceded to. Even his proposal to withdraw from practice for five years, in order to study the subject without interruption, secured him no better reception. Moreover, the medical press, with the exception of the *Lancet* and a very few others, denounced Marshall Hall virulently. In one number of a quarterly journal no fewer than four articles attacked the discovery, one denying its originality while allowing it to be true, another denouncing Dr. Hall's views as new but not true. The long persistence of this opposition was almost incredible; for years one journal kept it up through every number; each step was disputed, and what was indisputable was depreciated. "Ancient works were disinterred in the vain hope of robbing him of his originality. 'Complete anticipations' were exultingly announced. On the one hand, he was accused of stealing his ideas from old writers; on the other, contemporaries started up and claimed the discovery as theirs; while some combated its truth, and never ceased cavilling."

While the Royal Society refused him any honours, and in 1847, ten years after the last paper, rejected another which he sent in, detailing an experimental research on the relation of galvanism to the nervous and muscular tissues, Marshall Hall never ceased his investigations. He did not, however, like some few men of originality, disdain to reply to attacks. He was even anxious to refute any and every mis-statement made about him and his work, his view being: " It would not be truthful in me; and why should I fear to declare the truth?" "I appeal from the first half of the nineteenth century to the second." "I am as certain of the truth of what I have advanced, as I am of my own existence." But while his opponents denounced him as irritable and thin-skinned, it is testified of him that his temper was never affected; neither petulance nor gloom clouded his life; he never wrote an anonymous unfavourable review. "Nothing delighted his benevolent heart," says his widow, "more than to praise others, when he could conscientiously do so; and never can I forget the sparkle of his eye and his pleasant smile when he had written something in favour of any professional brother."

Practice now flowed in upon Dr. Hall. His researches gave him an insight into diseases and disorders of the nervous system which no one had as yet approached. Large numbers of patients came to consult him personally, or sent for him without the intervention of a general practitioner. Dr. Russell Reynolds says that his "New Memoir on the Nervous System," 1843, described with remarkable ingenuity the mechanism of the convulsive paroxysm, and of many other affections assuming a paroxysmal type. "To Dr. Marshall Hall is due the merit of having rescued the obscure class of convulsive affections from a region of utter unintelligibility. The action of strychnia as a spinal excitant, or, in small doses, as a spinal tonic; the direction—general, regiminal, and medical—of the epileptic patient,

in order to avoid all the excitants of convulsive action;
the recommendation of tracheotomy in laryngismal
epilepsy; and the simple but beautiful ' Ready Method
in Asphyxia,' were among the later efforts of Dr.
Hall's great genius. . . . The two prominent features of
his treatment were simplicity and perseverance. We
have seen numerous cases in which his administration
of simple aperients, together with strictly regiminal
measures, had wrought extraordinary cures; and we
know of previously paraplegic men, now well, who
under his direction took strychnia for much longer
than a year; and of so-called epileptics who slowly
recovered from the most frightful combination of
symptoms, while kept by Dr. Hall for sixteen or
eighteen months under the influence of mercury."
Even under the heaviest strain of practice he found
time to continue his researches, and to publish his
experience. In 1845 and 1846 appeared two small
volumes of "Practical Observations and Suggestions in
Medicine," in which a great number of medical subjects
were treated in so concise and telling a way that they
were immediately welcomed by a large class of readers.
A chapter on the use of the Alcoholic Lotion in Phthisis
Pulmonalis is said to have been the means of saving
many lives; another on "the Temper Disease" is most
interesting to the student of human nature as well as
of medicine.

A friend, Mr. Henry Gregory, of Herne Hill, who
had much professional and friendly intercourse with

Dr. Hall, says of him : " In debate or conversational argument nothing seemed to escape his penetration. His minuteness in bringing out little things which others thought not of, was remarkable; with one little atom, so to speak, a light would shine forth from him so brilliantly that I could only sit and admire his remarkable mental gifts. He was a great man and a genius, and, like all the truly great, made no parade. . . . He was the educator of the intellect; his domain was pure scientific research. The earnest activity of his mind made him proceed, and every advance he made was a clearing away of error and an establishment of truth. . . . In emergencies he was both prompt and cautious; when anxious excitement surrounded him, it did not disturb his judgment. In dangerous and difficult cases he was always calm. His deep sense of duty and responsibility was unbending." There is a universal concurrence of testimony as to his great success in gaining his patients' confidence ; young and old looked with delight for his visits. He would always direct the responsible nurse most precisely, and endeavour by every possible device to secure that his special treatment should be carried out. His searching and pointed questions not unfrequently discovered "hidden seizures," as he called them, which had been totally unsuspected or uncomprehended by patients or friends. His power of devising a remedy is amusingly illustrated by his prescription to an indolent lady that she was to walk daily to the Serpentine from her home, and dip her finger in it. The desirability of healthy mental occupation, and the encouragement of happiness and pleasing customs generally, were favourite subjects of his injunctions. Sympathy and kindliness shone through his whole manner. A Scotch minister said to him : "You place your soul in the stead of your patient's soul." But he abhorred all coaxing and wheedling; he hated cant. He would not lower his own lofty sense of independence by anything approaching to it. One might have supposed so sympathetic a nature would have been compliant; but his spirit and dignity were consistent with and equal to his sympathy. It was but another phase of his noble character that he could attend the poor and the needy middle-class without allowing or causing them to feel the slightest difference between themselves and the rich.

This was the great physician who could never find a post as physician in any London hospital. His medical teaching was almost entirely confined to the schools that were outside the close circle of the hospital schools. In 1834–6 he lectured on medicine at the Aldersgate School, and then joined the Webb Street School (that of the Graingers), taking a similar post. He also gave lectures for two years at "Sydenham College," established near University College. But the exertion of lecturing concurrently at these two was too much for his voice, and he could not complete his course in 1839. In 1842–6 he gave lectures on nervous diseases, at St. Thomas's Hospital Medical

School. In these he illustrated many points by remarkable diagram portraits of paralytic patients. His lectures were given extemporaneously after careful preparation, and delivered extremely clearly, without any showiness. When lecturing at a school un-attached to a hospital he would invite his pupils by turns to breakfast at his house, that they might then see some of his poorer patients, and go over their cases with him. One instance of his thoughtfulness for his pupils is enough to mark out any man from among his fellows. A student was confined to his room for three or four weeks by illness, and Dr. Hall came regularly to his lodgings to give him a *resumé* of his lecture, and of what followed it. No wonder that an affectionate feeling bound his class to him, and that no lecturer ever was more attentively followed. The instances of the affection and regard displayed in various ways between him and his pupils are among the most interesting records in medical biography.*

Though he had been denied the Fellowship of the College of Physicians until 1841, Marshall Hall was at last fully recognised by the College in being appointed to deliver the Gulstonian lectures in 1842, and the Croonian in 1850, 1, and 2. In these courses, which were largely attended, he fully explained his views and discoveries on the nervous system and nervous diseases, as well as on general medical treatment.

* Memorials of Marshall Hall, by his widow, 1861.

They were published later, in the form of " Synopses "
of each course, in quarto.

Notwithstanding his aversion to anything like strife
in medical politics, Marshall Hall took a prominent
part in the formation of the British Medical Association,
and was at once elected on its Council, and delivered
the oration on Medical Reform in 1840. He was in
his true place in every philanthropic scheme that
needed medical advocacy. The open railway carriages
were doomed when he denounced them as dangerous
to health; inhuman flogging of soldiers was evidently
condemned when he expounded the character of the
injuries inflicted on the cutaneous nerves, and the
degree of shock to the heart. He even wrote on the
Higher Powers of Numbers, in the *Mechanics' Magazine*,
and took an interest in devising new forms of con-
jugation for Greek nouns and verbs. He strongly
advocated a new Pharmacopœia, based on the decimal
system. He suggested in a pamphlet as early as 1850
new works for the sewerage of the Thames, developing
his ideas more elaborately in 1852 and 1856. Many
of his views and plans have since been adopted: others
must and will still be carried out if London is to be
properly and healthily drained.

It is not to be imagined that Hall was so absorbed
in study and practice that he could not take recreation.
No one enjoyed more than he the pleasure of travelling, the tonic of the open air, the change to the Continent, a tour to America; and he rigorously took

these, and enjoyed himself with the *abandon* of a
child. His delight in splendid scenery was extreme;
and he gratified his taste, in season, by tours extending very widely over Europe. His visit to America
was specially undertaken in 1853 with the object of
studying slavery by personal observation. In New
York and other cities he gave lectures by request
illustrative of his discoveries. From Quebec to New
Orleans, and even the Havana, his fame had preceded
him, and he was feted and listened to with as much
ceremony and enthusiasm as his retiring nature could
be prevailed upon to endure. At the Havana he
lectured in French for two hours, and the medical
students of the city visited him again and again, thirst-
ing for information at first hand. Dr. and Mrs. Hall
returned to England in April 1854; and very soon
after he published his little volume on "The Two-
fold Slavery of the United States." The subject was
one which most deeply interested Marshall Hall's
philosophical and religious mind; and it is significant
of the depth of his philosophy that he was far-seeing
enough to be certain that unprepared abolition would
be far from a perfect boon for the slave, while yet he
regarded the continuation of slavery as wicked and
degrading, financially ruinous, and tending to generate
wars. His remedies were first, education; second, the
appointment of fair task-work; third, the privilege of
over-work, to be paid for, and the payments accumulated
till freedom could be purchased with the aid of pro-

portionate additions by the Federal and States' Govern-
ments. Whether his plan could ever have been worked
out will now never be known. That many of the evils
he foresaw have followed persistence in slavery and
sudden abolition is matter of certainty.

Marshall Hall's physical frame had been overtaxed
by his exertions and struggles, and he became in-
creasingly liable to severe laryngitis. Taking another
continental trip in the winter of 1854–5, he showed
his vivid intellectual energy by applying himself at
Rome to the study of Hebrew. He engaged a Rabbi
to teach him, and when awake at night or at early
dawn, he worked at his new study with the zeal of
a tripos candidate, and never did a pupil make more
rapid progress. He ascended Vesuvius during the
eruption of May 1855, a serious undertaking for a
man of sixty-five. At Paris, in the summer, he wrote
in three months a work in French, detailing his investigations on the spinal system, dedicated to M.
Flourens, who had always shown the most generous
appreciation of his labours as constituting a great
epoch in physiology. Louis, the great physician, and
his wife, were equally warm in their appreciation of
and attachment to him. On December 5, 1855,
Marshall Hall was elected a corresponding member of
the French Academy of Science, by 39 votes out of 41.

On returning to England towards the end of 1855,
Marshall Hall's mind fastened with characteristic
eagerness on a new subject, suggested by reading the

Humane Society's "Rules to Restore the Apparently
Drowned." He remarked: "There is nothing in the
treatment to restore respiration." He at once thought
out the question in the light of his researches on the
physiology of respiration, and when he had mentally
devised his system of restoration, proceeded to make
experiments to test them. Hitherto it had been
believed that it was useless to attempt to restore those
who had been immersed three or four minutes. He said
to the Secretary of the Humane Society: "If we take
this for granted, we shall do nothing; surely it is
worth while to make the effort to restore after a longer
period." His plan for producing artificial respiration,
by turning the body first on the face, then on the
side, and repeating the motion for a quarter of an
hour, making equable pressure on the back of the
chest when in the prone position, removing it when
rotating on to the side, is known all over the world
as the Marshall Hall method, and has saved thousands
of lives. Numerous details are added to increase the
efficiency of the treatment. But the Humane Society
looked coldly on the novel plan, and long persisted
in ignoring it. The National Lifeboat Institution
wisely adopted it; the medical profession received it
with acclamation; it was applied to the revival of
still-born infants, and the restoration of those in
danger of dying from asphyxia from other causes than
drowning. At the same time when Palmer's trial for
poisoning was occurring, Dr. Hall drew attention to

the facility with which the presence of strychnia could be proved by administering any suspected matter to young frogs, which would be affected by the five-thousandth part of a grain of strychnia.

But he now began to succumb to the effects of his long-continued malady in the throat. Expectoration of blood became more frequent, difficulty of swallowing increased; at times he was near absolute starvation, and his sufferings were horrible, but his patience and resignation marvellous. After months of terrible illness, during which his cheerfulness never left him, he died on the 11th August 1857, of ulceration of the upper part of the gullet and windpipe. During his illness his mind was as active as ever, he wrote continually his new ideas, and worked out to fuller ends his former discoveries. Throughout he was especially bright and affectionate to all little children ; the manner in which he entered into children's delights was most exquisite to witness. His Christian faith was unclouded; as he said, religion was to him the principal thing. In the simplicity, beauty, and happiness of his character he resembled Sir Charles Bell, of whom he was the true successor.

CHAPTER X.

SIR BENJAMIN BRODIE AND SIR WILLIAM LAW-
RENCE, TWO GREAT PRACTICAL SURGEONS.

THE influence of heredity and of association and con-
nexion with talented persons is well illustrated in
the case of Sir Benjamin Brodie. His paternal grandfather, Alexander Brodie, was a native of Banffshire,
who came to London as a humble adventurer and
almost as a Jacobite refugee. He married a daughter
of a physician named Shaw, of similar Jacobite family
and connexions. Brodie became an army clothier, and
one of his daughters, who married Dr. Denman, the
eminent obstetric physician, was the mother of Lord
Denman. Margaret and Sophia, the twin daughters of
Dr. Denman, married—the former Sir Richard Croft,
who attended the Princess Charlotte at her death in
1817, the latter Dr. Matthew Baillie, the eminent
physician, and nephew of John Hunter. The army
clothier's wife was herself a woman of considerable
abilities, and it was said that there was royal blood in
the family.

The father of Sir Benjamin was educated at Char-
terhouse and at Oxford. As a boy he was patronised

by the first Lord Holland, and spent much time at
Holland House. A warm attachment existed between
them, in which Charles James Fox shared. When
Lord Holland died in 1774, he directed by will that
Mr. Brodie, who had taken holy orders, should have
the next presentation to whichever of his livings first
became vacant. This desire was soon fulfilled, and
Winterslow in Wiltshire became the home of the
Brodies. The Rev. Mr. Brodie married in 1775 a
daughter of Mr. Collins, a banker at Salisbury; and of
this marriage Benjamin Collins Brodie was the third
son, having been born in 1783.

Sir Benjamin in his "Autobiography" gives a pleasing
picture of his father, a man of sound classical knowledge, great energy, minute acquaintance with parish-
ioners, and devotion to his parochial duties. Notwithstanding his wife's considerable fortune, Mr. Brodie
found he could not afford to send all his sons to public
schools, and he consequently determined to educate
them himself. An elder sister who joined the brothers
at lessons became no mean proficient in classics. Under
the strict discipline of their father the children grew
up in the habit of methodical study, and Sir Benjamin
records that idleness even for a day was always irksome to him in after life, and he had little inclina-
tion for any pursuit without a definite ulterior object.
Seven miles distant from Salisbury, the family learned
to be self-dependent for interest of all kinds, and
their solitude was little varied except by occasional

visits of cousins, such as Lord Denman, who was for a
year a resident pupil with Mr. Brodie after leaving
Eton, and a few others, one of whom was afterwards
Dr. Maton, a well-known London physician, and (Sir)
John Stoddart, afterwards Chief Justice at Malta.
Vigour of character was shown markedly when in 1798
the brothers raised a company of volunteers on the
alarm of a French invasion. The eldest at nineteen
received a commission as captain, while Benjamin, only
fourteen, was appointed ensign. Great pains were
bestowed on the drill of this company, and the officers
expended their pay in entertaining the men in a great
barn; and the influence already possessed by the
youths was evident in the maintenance and increase of
the numbers of the corps and the attention paid to drill.
The eldest brother, Peter, became a distinguished con-
veyancing barrister. The second was a local banker,
proprietor of a newspaper, and represented Salisbury
in three Parliaments.

As he drew towards adult age, Brodie read extensively in science and philosophy and general literature.
In the autumn of 1801, the medical profession having
been chosen for him, he went to London without any
special bent towards the occupation in which he was
destined to shine so conspicuously. He gives it as his
opinion, in after years, that those who succeed best in
professions are those who have embarked in them not
from irresistible prepossession but perhaps from some
accidental circumstance, and persevere in their course as

a matter of duty, or because they have nothing better to do. "They often feel their new pursuit to be unattractive enough in the beginning; but as they go on, and acquire knowledge, and find that they obtain some degree of credit, the case is altered; and from that time they become every day more interested in what they are about:"—a great encouragement to the vast majority of students who do not feel the stimulus and inspiration of genius.

During his first season in London, young Brodie attended Abernethy's course on Anatomy, and to his influence may be attributed the choice of surgery as his special vocation. "He kept up our attention," says Brodie, "so that it never flagged, and what he told us could not be forgotten." One of his earliest friendships was that which he formed with William Lawrence as a fellow-student. This continued unbroken throughout life, and though they might be regarded as rivals, no jealousy ever arose between them. But Brodie was more at home with his non-medical friends, his elder brother with whom he lodged, Denman, Merivale, Wray, Stoddart, Gifford (afterwards Lord Gifford), and Maton. The latter had established in London the Academical Society, as a sort of transplant from Oxford, and Brodie was here introduced to Lord Glenelg and his brother Robert Grant, Francis Horner, Dr. Bateman, and "a young Scotchman of uncouth appearance," afterwards Lord Campbell. Before this Society Brodie read papers on metaphysical enquiries and on the

principles of science, showing his philosophical bent.
Berkeley was the author who influenced him most
powerfully, from his clear reasoning and simple un-
affected perspicuous style, terms which are specially
appropriate to Brodie's own writing.

In 1802 Wilson's lectures on anatomy at Great Windmill Street were Brodie's main professional pabulum.
" I was naturally very clumsy in the use of my hands,"
he says, "and it was only by taking great pains with
myself that I became at all otherwise." In the spring
of 1803 he became a pupil of Home (afterwards Sir
Everard) at St. George's Hospital, continuing also his
anatomical studies. He ultimately became Sir Everard's
assistant both in the hospital and in private practice.
From this connection, however, he derived little pecuniary profit, but by aiding Home in his researches in
comparative anatomy and physiology he gained decided benefit. In 1805, however, Brodie became demonstrator in Wilson's anatomical school. He was introduced to Sir Joseph Banks, and through him to the
best scientific men of the day. Could there be more
favourable conditions for progress, or circumstances more
unlike these of chilling seclusion and neglect which
have so often hindered and overshadowed men of
merit ?

Brodie continued to demonstrate, and from 1809 to
lecture at Great Windmill Street, until in 1812 (Sir)
Charles Bell became principal lecturer there. In 1808
he was appointed assistant surgeon at St. George's

Hospital, by Home's influence, and in reality did the work of a full surgeon almost from that date. Private practice he scarcely attempted, his hands being full of anatomical and hospital work. Robert Keate and Brodie were at the hospital daily, and superintended everything; there was never an urgent case that they did not visit in the evening. This surgical experience was at once turned to advantage by Wilson, who asked Brodie to join him in lecturing on surgery. From 1809 onward for nearly twenty years, Brodie gave this course of lectures, and had a good attendance of students; besides which he lectured on surgery at St. George's Hospital till 1840. In 1809 he took a house in Sackville Street and received three private pupils, and in 1810 felt justified, from the increase of his means, in engaging in physiological enquiries, stimulated by Bichat's researches. He was elected into the Royal Society in 1810; and in the same and following winter communicated to the Society two valuable papers, one "On the Influence of the Brain on the Action of the Heart and the Generation of Animal Heat;" and the other "On the Effects produced by certain Vegetable Poisons." The former was given as the Croonian Lecture in 1810. These papers, though largely superseded by recent investigations, were quite remarkable for their time, and for the first he was awarded the Copley Medal in 1811, which had never before been given to so young a man.

It is worth noting that a medal was awarded by the

Royal Society to the second Sir Benjamin Brodie in 1850, for his investigations "on the chemical nature of wax." With the exception of the two Herschels, this is the only instance in which father and son have received this honour. The most noted, perhaps, of Brodie's physiological papers was one on the influence of the nervous system on the production of animal heat, published in 1812. He concluded that an animal with the nervous centres removed, or with their functions suspended by narcotic poison, lost its power of generating heat, even though the action of the lungs was kept up by artificial respiration. Brodie used the then little known woorara poison brought by Dr. Bancroft from Guiana, to produce suspension of the nervous action. In after life increase of practice left little time for further physiological research.

At length Brodie married (in 1816) Ann, the third daughter of Serjeant Sellon, his bride being only nineteen. This was in every way a happy marriage; and Sir Benjamin always warmly recognised his wife's excellent moral training of their children. In the year of their marriage Brodie's professional income from fees and lectures amounted to £1530. For some years he had paid special attention to diseases of the joints, which were then very ill understood; and in 1819 he published his classical work "On the Pathology and Surgery of Diseases of the Joints." He clearly distinguished between diseases of the various tissues of which joints are composed; and also between hysterical, neuralgic, and merely local diseases. Many limbs, in which no disease could be found after removal, were at that time removed merely because pain was felt in them. A story told in the *Lancet* on this subject is worth reproducing.

"Late one evening a person came into our office, and asked to see the Editor of the *Lancet.* On being introduced to our sanctum, he placed a bundle upon the table, from which he proceeded to extract a very fair and symmetrical lower extremity, and which had evidently belonged to a woman. 'There!' said he, 'is there anything the matter with that leg? Did you ever see a handsomer? What ought the man to be done with who cut it off?' On having the meaning of those interrogatories put before us, we found that it was the leg of the wife of our evening visitor. He had been accustomed to admire the lady's leg and foot, of the perfection of which she was, it appeared, fully conscious. A few days before, he had excited her anger, and they had quarrelled violently, upon which she left the house, declaring she would be revenged on him, and that he should never see the objects of his admiration again. The next thing he heard of her was that she was a patient in —— Hospital, and had had her leg amputated. She had declared to the surgeons that she suffered intolerable pain in the knee, and had begged to have the limb removed—a petition the surgeons complied with, and thus became the instrument of her absurd and self-torturing revenge upon her husband."

Brodie may now be regarded as firmly established in
public favour. His income in 1819 exceeded that of
the preceding year by £1000. He enjoyed the intimate
acquaintance of Lord and Lady Holland, and the sunshine of their friendship had its strong influence on
practice. In 1819 Brodie removed to Savile Row, and
in the same year was appointed to succeed Lawrence
as Professor of Comparative Anatomy and Physiology
at the College of Surgeons. In this capacity he lectured
for four years, delivering new and original matter each
time. They constituted a frightful addition to his
labours, and he only completed them by taking many
hours from needed sleep. He records, however, that
few things contributed more to his improvement than
the composition of his lectures, and the habit of recording his knowledge and thoughts. It enabled him to
detect his own deficiencies, and to avoid hasty conclusions, and taught him to be less conceited of his own
opinions.

An important branch of modern surgery may be
said to have had its rise in an operation first performed
by Brodie. Now-a-days subcutaneous operations, in
which the slightest possible opening is made in the
skin, and frequently considerable incisions or other
interferences are made beneath it, are very common,
and the procedure is of the greatest importance in
orthopædic surgery and the relief of muscular and
tendinous contractions of various kinds. Brodie
first performed a subcutaneous operation for the relief

of varicose veins of the legs in 1814, and several similar cases were published by him in the seventh volume of the " Medico-Chirurgical Transactions." If no other operative improvement of great moment is associated with Brodie's name, it is not that he has not left his mark on that department of practice, but rather that he has been the introducer of innumerable minor improvements. In particular, he was notable in devising improvements in surgical instruments and apparatus.

In 1821, Brodie was called in to attend George IV., who very much wished him to perform the operation which in deference to Lord Liverpool was entrusted to Sir Astley Cooper. Brodie remained ever after a favourite with George IV. and attended him frequently during his last illness, going to Windsor every evening, and visiting the King at six in the morning and remaining with him for an hour or two before returning to London. When William IV. came to the throne, Brodie was appointed Serjeant Surgeon, and soon after received a baronetcy. He had now for some years been at the head of his profession, having succeeded to Sir Astley's place on his retirement in 1828. In 1823 his income was already £6500; for many years his practice brought him £10,000 and sometimes £11,000 a year. This was a very remarkable income considering the small proportion of it that was derived from operations. Much the greatest part he took in single guinea fees, and thus it is seen how much his opinion was valued in surgical cases. Indeed he often, especially after his retirement from St. George's Hospital in 1840, refused to perform important operations to which he felt no special attraction. But his abiding popularity and influence is shown by the fact that his total receipts from fees, from first to last, considerably exceeded Sir Astley's. He used to say that he had always kept in mind the saying of William Scott (afterwards Lord Stowell) to his brother John (subsequently Lord Eldon), " John, always keep the Lord Chancellorship in view, and you will be sure to get it in the end:" and a similar aim and distinction were Brodie's.

Meanwhile, the public interest was by no means lost sight of in private practice. To Brodie is largely due the merit of having put a stop to the career of St. John Long, the fashionable medical impostor. Sir Benjamin was one afternoon on his way to visit a friend at Hampstead, when he was called in to see a Miss Cashin. Finding an enormous slough on her back, caused by Long's treatment, he exclaimed, " Why, this is no better than murder!" The lady died, and on the strength of Sir Benjamin's expressions, an inquest was held, followed by the trial and condemnation of Long. Yet such was the strength of the fashionable partisanship in favour of the impostor, that the judge, Mr. Justice Park, merely fined him £250, which he at once paid. A second trial in another case, where death had ensued upon his treatment, ended in a verdict of acquittal.

In 1834 Sir Benjamin succeeded to the first vacancy

that occurred, after his appointment as Serjeant Surgeon, in the Court of Examiners of the College of Surgeons; this was by prescription due to his court office. He found this duty very irksome, and he resigned it when a new charter, which he had been largely instrumental in obtaining, no longer granted this privilege to the Serjeant Surgeon.

In 1839 and '40 Sir Benjamin was President of the Royal Medical and Chirurgical Society, and here again he shone. In addition to his own most valuable contributions, he excelled in drawing out others. His attendance was most diligent; his mind was never at a loss for something interesting to say; he stimulated discussion when an opposite precedent had been established; and to him a very large share of the Society's prosperity was due. Of course the Presidency of the Royal College of Surgeons fell to his lot. When the General Medical Council was established, Sir Benjamin was by common consent called to the Presidency; and in 1858 he received a still more remarkable honour in being called to the Presidency of the Royal Society, which office he held with dignity and wisdom till 1861. It is impossible for us here to record all the important offices Brodie filled, nor all the valuable communications he made to learned societies and various journals. Fortunately his charming autobiography is very accessible, being published separately as well as in the excellent collection of works, in three vols., 1865, edited by Mr. Charles Hawkins.

It is easily imagined that Brodie's long course of labour could only have been sustained by a strong constitution. He was not altogether robust, but by careful management succeeded in preserving excellent health. In 1834, while in the Isle of Wight, he fell from a pony and dislocated his right shoulder joint, which long after became diseased. In July 1860 his sight became impaired, and he ultimately submitted to excision of the iris of both eyes by Mr. (now Sir William) Bowman. Later, he was operated on for cataract; but all efforts to preserve good sight were futile. In July 1862 he began to suffer in his right shoulder, and finally died of cancerous disease in that joint on October 21st, 1862. He was buried at Betchworth, Surrey, in which parish the estate, Broome Park, which he had purchased, is situated.

The *Lancet* said of him, " It is true praise of Sir Benjamin Brodie to say, that he was more distinguished as a physician-surgeon than as an operating-surgeon. His vocation was more to heal limbs than to remove them. His imagination had never been dazzled by the brilliancy of the knife, to any great operative display. He was, however, always a most steady and successful operator: lightness of hand, caution without timidity, never-failing coolness, and fertility of resources, were his distinguishing characteristics. He made no secret of his opinion, that the operative part of surgery was not its highest part. Diagnosis had always been his great strength, and his opinion was, therefore, always deeply

valued by the profession and the public. We believe
his heart was with hospital, rather than private
practice, but in almost all cases men are more fond of
their early occupations than of those which come afterwards. As a teacher, he was always distinguished for
the value of the matter he had to communicate. Those
who heard him in the early part of his career say that
he was then energetic rather than polished; that he
appeared to struggle with the weight and mass of facts
he had stored up in his mind. But, in later years,
his delivery was fluent and perfect. No man in his
profession could deliver himself more readily or more
elegantly than Sir Benjamin Brodie."

Dr. Babington, President of the Royal Medical and
Chirurgical Society, thus characterised Brodie :—" As a
practical surgeon Sir Benjamin Brodie attained a
success far beyond that of most of his contemporaries,
and this he seems to have owed, not to personal appearance or manner, not to eccentricity, not to an unusual
degree of courtesy on the one hand, or of bluntness or
brusquery on the other, but to the legitimate influence
of a high order of intellect, thoroughly devoted to the
practical application of the stores of surgical knowledge
acquired by his assiduity and experience—to the sound,
well-considered, and decided opinions which his patients
were sure to obtain from him, and to the confidence
which his high religious principles and his strict
morality inspired. . . . For myself, I can only say that
I never knew a more single-minded and upright

character, one more free from affectation or presumption, who expected less deference or deserved more, or
who more completely impressed me with a belief that
the main object of his efforts, that which was always
uppermost on his mind, was, wholly irrespective of
self, to benefit those by whom he was consulted."

Dr. (now Sir Henry) Acland has given in the
Proceedings of the Royal Society perhaps the best
survey of Brodie's character and work:—"Neither as
scientific man, nor as surgeon, nor as author was he
so remarkable as he appears when viewed as he was—
a complete man necessarily engaged in various callings.
It was impossible to see him acting in any capacity
without instinctively feeling that there he would do his
duty, and do it well. Nor could he be imagined in a
false position. A gentleman, according to his own
definition of that word, he did to others that which he
would desire to be done to him, respecting them as he
respected himself. Simple in his manners, he gained
confidence at once; accustomed to mix with the poorest
in the hospital and with the noblest in their private
abodes, he sympathised with the better qualities of
each,—valued all, and despised nothing but moral
meanness. Though as a boy he was retiring and
modest, he was happy in the company of older persons,
and, as he grew older, loved in his turn to help the
young. 'I hear you are ill,' he wrote once in the
zenith of his life to a hospital student of whom he did
not then know much; 'no one will take better care of

you than I; come to my country house till you are
well;' and the student stayed there two months. He
was thought by some reserved—he was modest; by
others hasty—he valued time, and could not give to
trifles that which belonged to real suffering; he was
sometimes thought impatient, when his quick glance
had already told him more than the patient could
either describe or understand. Unconscious of self, of
strong common-sense, confident of his ground or not
entering thereon, seeing in every direction, modest,
just, sympathetic, he lived for one great end, the
lessening of disease. For this object no labour was too
great, no patience too long, no science too difficult.
He felt indeed his happiness to be in a life of exertion.
As a professional man he valued science because it so
often points the way to that which is practically useful
to many; but as a scientific man his one object was
the truth, which he pursued for its own sake, wholly
irrespective of any other reward which might or might
not follow on discovery. He had not the common
faults of common men, for he had not their objects,
nor their instinct for ease, nor their prejudices; though
he became rich, he had not unduly sought riches;
though he was greatly distinguished, he had not desired
fame; he was beloved, not having courted popularity.
What he was himself, that he allowed other men to be,
till he found them otherwise. He saw weak points in
his profession, but he saw them as the débris from the
mountains of knowledge and wisdom, of benevolence

302 TWO GREAT PRACTICAL SURGEONS.

and of self-denial, of old traditional skill ever growing and always purifying,—those eternal structures on
which are founded true surgery and medicine. If ever
he was bitter in society, it was when they were under-
valued; if ever sarcastic, it was when the ignorant
dared presume to judge them.

"A light is thus thrown on his even career of uniform
progress. Training his powers from youth upwards,
by linguistic and literary studies, by scientific pursuits,
by the diligent practice of his art, by mixing with men,
he brought to bear on the multifarious questions which
come before a great master of healing, a mind alike
accustomed to acquire and to communicate, a temper
made gentle by considerate kindness, a tact that
became all but unerring from his perfect integrity.
He saw that every material science conduces to the
well-being of man; he would countenance all, and yet
be distracted by none. He knew the value of worldly
influence, of rank, of station, when rightly used; he
sought none, deferred excessively to none; but he
respected all who, having them, used them wisely,
and accepted what came to himself unasked, gave
his own freely to all who needed, and sought help
from no one but for public ends. . . . . Those who
knew him only as a man of business, would little
suspect the playful humour which sparkled by his
fireside, the fund of anecdote—the harmless wit, the
simple pleasures of his country walk.

"In the quality of his mind he was not unlike

the most eminent of his contemporaries, Arthur Duke of Wellington. Those who did not know him, and who do not appreciate the power requisite to make such a master in medicine as he was, may be surprised at the comparison. Yet our great soldier might have accepted the illustration without dissatisfaction. Whatever art Brodie undertook, if he has been correctly drawn, he would have entirely mastered. The self-discipline of the strongest man can effect no more. The care with which the two men compassed every detail, and surveyed every bearing of a large question, the quiet good sense, the steadiness of purpose, the readiness of wide professional knowledge in critical emergencies, were in each alike. The public and his profession esteemed Brodie as the first in his art."

WILLIAM LAWRENCE was born at Cirencester in July 1783, his father having practised as a surgeon in that town for many years. After being educated at a classical school near Gloucester, young Lawrence was apprenticed in February 1799 to the celebrated Abernethy, in whose house he went to reside. In after years, when lecturing before the College of Surgeons for the first time, Lawrence spoke thus eloquently of his teacher:—"Having had the good fortune to be initiated in the profession by Mr. Abernethy, and to have lived for many years under his roof, I can assure you, with the greatest sincerity, that however highly the public may estimate the surgeon and the

philosopher, I have reason to speak still more highly
of the man and the friend; of the invariable kindness
which directed my early studies and pursuits, of the
disinterested friendship which has assisted every step
of my progress in life, and the benevolent and honourable feelings, the independent spirit and the liberal
conduct, which, while they dignify our profession,
win our love, and command our respect for genius and
knowledge, converting those precious gifts into instruments of the most extensive public good." Lawrence
proved himself so zealous a pupil that in the third year
of his apprenticeship, Abernethy appointed him to be
his demonstrator of anatomy, a post which he filled
for twelve years. Becoming a member of the College
of Surgeons in 1805, he was appointed Assistant
Surgeon to St. Bartholomew's Hospital in 1813, and
in the same year was elected F.R.S. Already in 1801
he had published a translation from the Latin of a
Description of the Arteries, by Murray, Professor at
Upsala. In 1806 he won a prize offered by the
College of Surgeons, for an essay on the Treatment of
Hernia. This essay when printed gained immediate
acceptance, and numerous editions were published.
Lawrence's contributions to anatomy and surgery now
followed rapidly, several appearing in the *Edinburgh
Medical and Physical Journal.* His observations on
Lithotomy showed the way to a revival of the true
system of operating laterally with the knife. In 1814
Lawrence was chosen surgeon to the Eye Hospital

at Moorfields, and in 1815 to the Royal Hospitals of Bridewell and Bethlehem. In the latter year he was selected for the Professorship of Anatomy and Physiology at the College of Surgeons, and hence arose one of the bitterest controversial tempests of the early part of this century.

Lawrence took occasion, in his first lectures in 1816, to criticise Abernethy's exposition of Hunter's theory of life, and to unfold views which seriously scandalised those who regarded life as a mysterious entity entirely separate from and above the material organism with which it is associated. These views were criticised by Abernethy in his "Physiological Lectures" in 1817, and Lawrence replied in 1818, in terms of sarcasm which made a serious breach between the master and his former pupil. Lawrence's lectures were published as "An Introduction to Comparative Anatomy and Physiology," 1816, and "Lectures on Physiology, Zoology, and the Natural History of Man," 1819. Having been accused by Abernethy and others "of perverting the honourable office intrusted to him, by the College of Surgeons, to the very unworthy design of propagating opinions detrimental to society, and of endeavouring to enforce them for the purpose of loosening those restraints on which the welfare of mankind depends," he used his eloquence unsparingly both to defend his position, and to repel the attacks made upon him. He was not more heretical than many of his predecessors, nor than a great many enlightened biologists of the present day. He regarded life as "the assemblage of all the functions. and the general result of their exercise. Thus organisation, vital properties, functions and life, are expressions related to each other; in which organisation is the instrument, vital properties the acting power, function the mode of action, and life the result." Again, "we find that the motion proper to living bodies, or in one word, Life, has its origin in that of their parents. From their parents they have received the vital impulse, and hence it is evident, that in the present state of things, life proceeds only from life; and there exists no other but that which has been transmitted from one living body to another by an uninterrupted succession."

Lawrence was virulently attacked, and his name associated with Tom Paine and Lord Byron as arch-heretics. A pamphlet of the year 1820 has the following title: "The Radical Triumvirate; or, Infidel Paine, Lord Byron, and Surgeon Lawrence colleaguing with the Patriotic Radicals to emancipate Mankind from all laws Human and Divine, with a plate engraved for their instruction: a Letter to John Bull from an Oxonian resident in London." The Christian Advocate in the University of Cambridge, the Rev. Thomas Rennell, among others, took up the task of controverting Lawrence's supposed materialism. The lectures on the comparative anatomy of man certainly put forward in a striking light many of Blumenbach's views, and showed that the literal accuracy of the early parts of Genesis was inconsistent with the facts of zoology and comparative anatomy. We might proceed further on this subject, but Lawrence himself prevented his successors from espousing his personal cause with ardour, for, being called upon to resign his position at Bridewell and Bethlehem, "he did not resign, but recanted; bought up all the copies of his work 'On the History of Man,' and sent them over to America." * Numerous modified and also spurious editions were sold. This conduct deprives him of a large share of our sympathy and respect. Had Lawrence, like Darwin or Huxley, maintained his opinions when most unpopular, he might have won a victory for sound science years before it actually was gained. If he had been the original discoverer of the truths he enunciated, and had bought them with his life's energy, he would scarcely have dropped them at the raging of a storm. But the glory was not to be his. He was tried in the balance and found wanting.

The early symptoms of disagreement between Abernethy and Lawrence extended to other members of the staff, and led to the establishment of the Aldersgate Street School of Medicine, where Lawrence lectured on surgery till 1828, when he succeeded to Abernethy's lectures on surgery at St. Bartholomew's. The Aldersgate School included able teachers, such as Tweedie, Clutterbuck, Roget, Tyrrell, and Davis, and had much

* *Lancet*, July 13, 1867. It has been since shown that Lawrence had nothing to do with the American speculation.

success.   Lawrence's connection with the Eye Infirmary
led him to become an authority on the surgery of the
eye.   He published in 1830 a treatise on the venereal
diseases of the eye, in 1833 a treatise on diseases of
the eye, besides other papers on this branch of practice.
Late in life he published, in 1863, his valuable "Lectures
on Surgery."   His smaller works and papers are too
numerous to mention.

As a student, Sir Benjamin Brodie describes William
Lawrence as already remarkable for his great powers
of acquirement, his industrious habits, and his immense
stores of information.   In later life he characterised
him as possessed of considerable powers of conversation, abounding in happy illustrations and not ill-
natured sarcasm.   "In public speaking," says Brodie,
" he is collected, has great command of language, and
uses it correctly.   In writing, his style is pure, free
from all affectation, yet in general not sufficiently
concise. . . That he is thoroughly acquainted with his
profession cannot be doubted."   But Sir Benjamin
does not attribute to him so much originality as erudition and industry.

It is in his relations to medical politics that the
conduct of William Lawrence is most open to question.
When the College of Surgeons was a close corporation,
he put himself at the head of a great agitation to
liberalise it.   An eloquent speech at the Freemasons'
Tavern in 1826 was one of the marked features of the
campaign, in which he joined heartily with the *Lancet* in

attacking the old-world system of the College. "But," says the *Lancet*, "the Council feared him, and elected him into their body. From that moment Mr. Lawrence became a conservative and an obstructive, and maintained that character to the close of his life. He not only deserted his former friends, but lost no opportunity of reviling them. . . Mr. Lawrence, during the long period that he was a member of the Council, and of the Court of Examiners, resolutely and consistently opposed every attempt that was made to improve the education and the status of the surgeon in general practice."

Lawrence was twice President of the College, and more than once delivered the Hunterian Oration. On the last of these occasions, in 1846, when a new charter had lately been obtained which failed to gratify the just aspirations of the members of the College, no one, it is said, could be persuaded to deliver the Hunterian Oration, till Lawrence, with characteristic polemic zeal, threw himself into the breach. A crowded audience, for the most part hostile, assembled; and Lawrence, instead of avoiding controversy, both defended and commended the action of the Council. A storm of indignation was excited, especially among those who had listened to his contrary deliverances twenty years before. But "the orator was imperturbable in the fiercest of the storm. He certainly displayed on that occasion his most extraordinary talents as an orator. When he had allowed his audience to exhaust their dissatisfaction at the sentiments which he had uttered, he concluded his address in a most masterly and eloquent peroration, which called forth the plaudits of the assembly."

" In arriving at a just estimation of the character of Sir W. Lawrence, it must be admitted," says the *Lancet,* "that in most of the higher qualities of the mind he was entitled to admiration. His talents were of the highest order, seldom surpassed in our profession. As a writer, his style was vigorous, clear, and convincing. As a lecturer, in manner, substance, and expression, he had no superior in the profession of our time, if we except Joseph Henry Green. As an operator, if not among the greatest, he is entitled to hold a high position. But it must be acknowledged that ' his principles were somewhat lax, his heart was somewhat hard.' We speak of him now merely in a public capacity, for in all the relations of private life he was most estimable and affectionate. Notwithstanding the low estimation in which he held surgeons in general practice, it is probable no pure surgeon of modern times ever had so large a general practice as himself. If they were only competent for the ' common exigencies of surgery,' he at all events thought himself able to treat every class of disease, whether medical or surgical."

In physical frame Lawrence was well developed and vigorous, above middle height, with a high forehead, a cold but keen blue eye, a classic nose, a large expressive mouth, and a firm chin of some size. He was always somewhat liable to loss of nerve power in the face or

in the lower limbs. In 1865 he began to become
enfeebled, and finally hemiplegia supervened, and a
second attack, at the Council Chamber of the College
of Surgeons, laid him by completely. But he remained
conscious till the last, dying on the 5th July 1867.
A bust of him adorns the rooms of the Medico-Chirurgical Society, and another is in the College of Surgeons.
A baronetcy was only conferred on him in the March
before his death. He had long been Surgeon Extraordinary to the Queen, and finally Serjeant Surgeon.
It has been said of him that he kept his appointments
as long as possible; but it may be answered that he
was full of vitality, and died in harness.

END OF VOL. I.